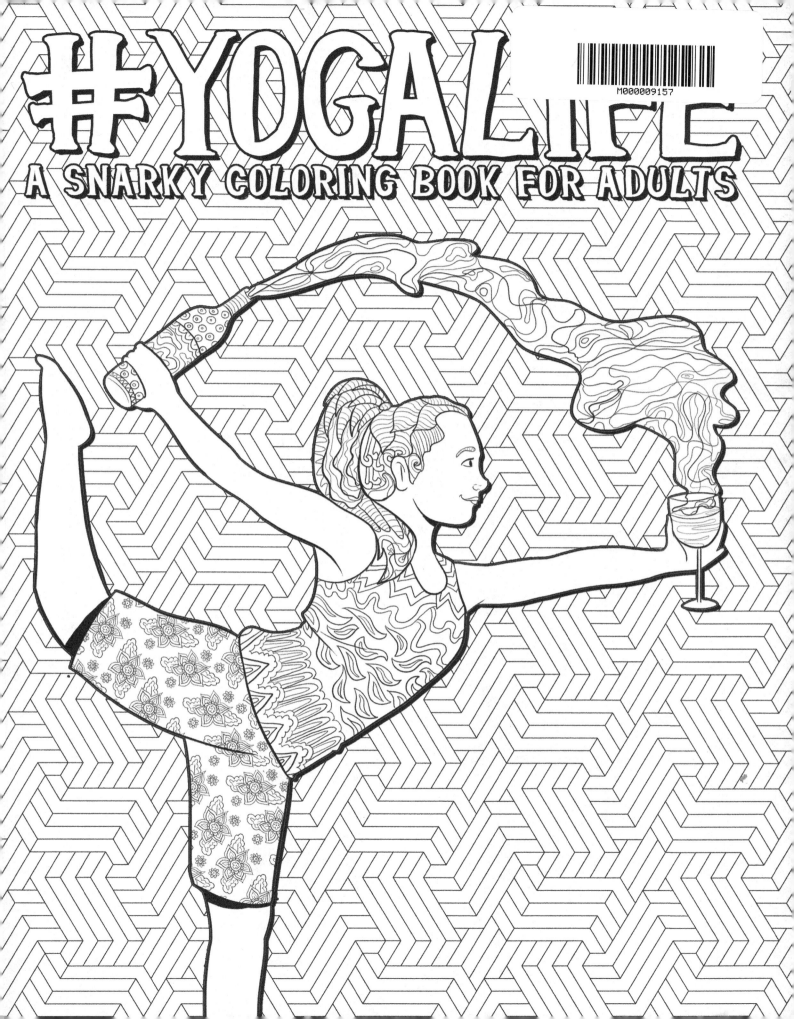

Want free goodies?
Email us at freebies@pbleu.com

@papeteriebleu

Papeterie Bleu

Shop our other books at
www.pbleu.com

Wholesale distribution through Ingram Content Group
www.ingramcontent.com/publishers/distribution/wholesale

For questions and customer service, email us at
support@pbleu.com

FREE PDF DOWNLOAD
OF THIS BOOK

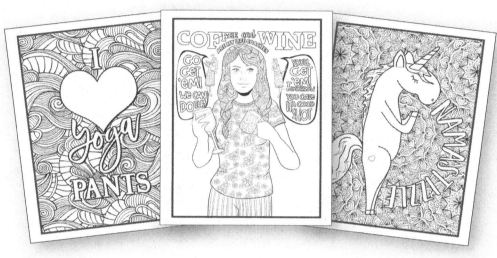

www.pbleu.com/yoga

YOUR DOWNLOAD CODE: YOGA373

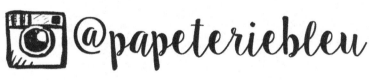 @papeteriebleu

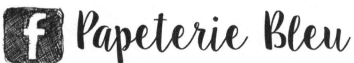 Papeterie Bleu

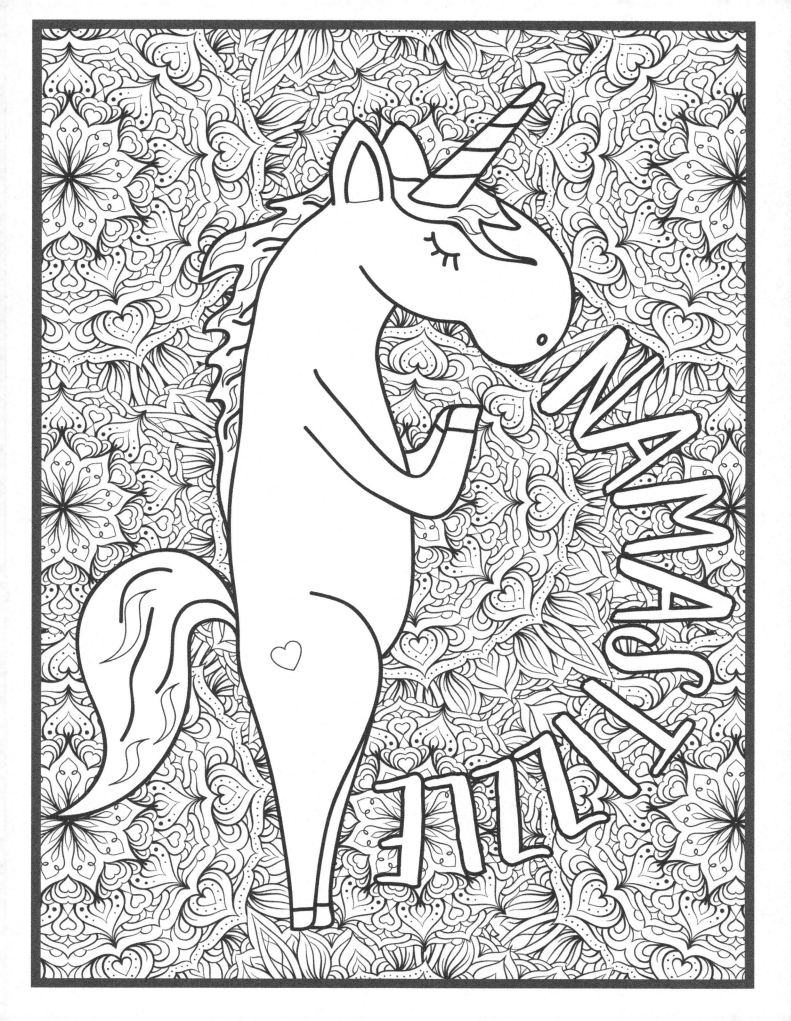

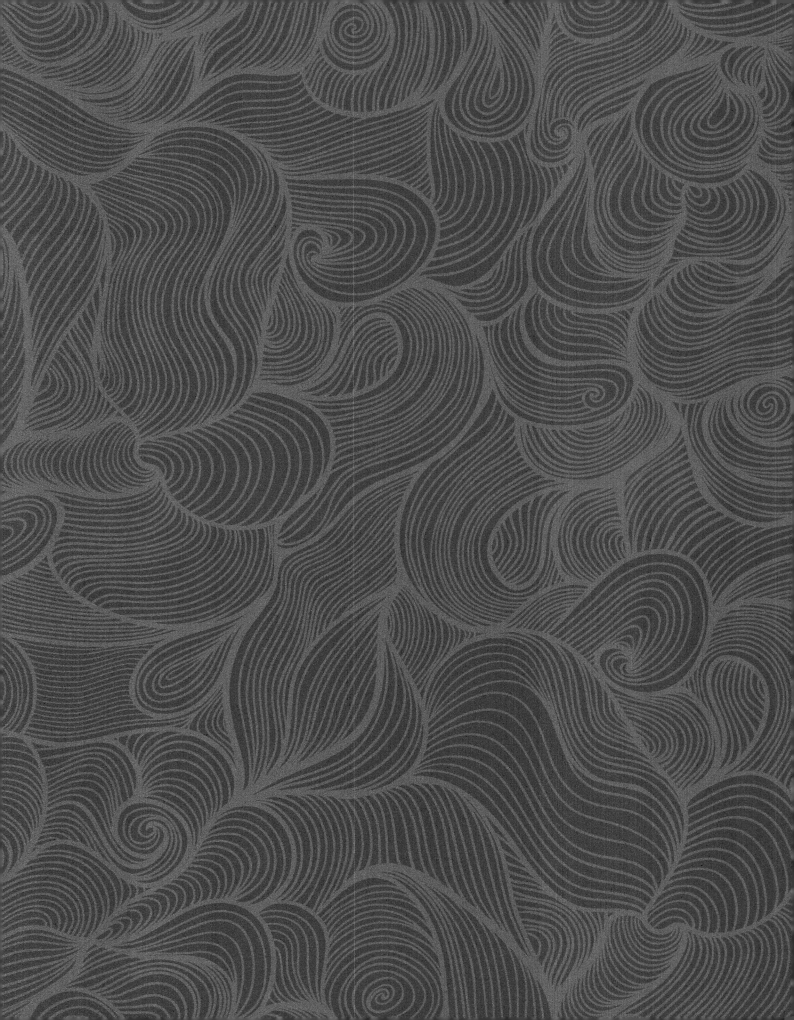

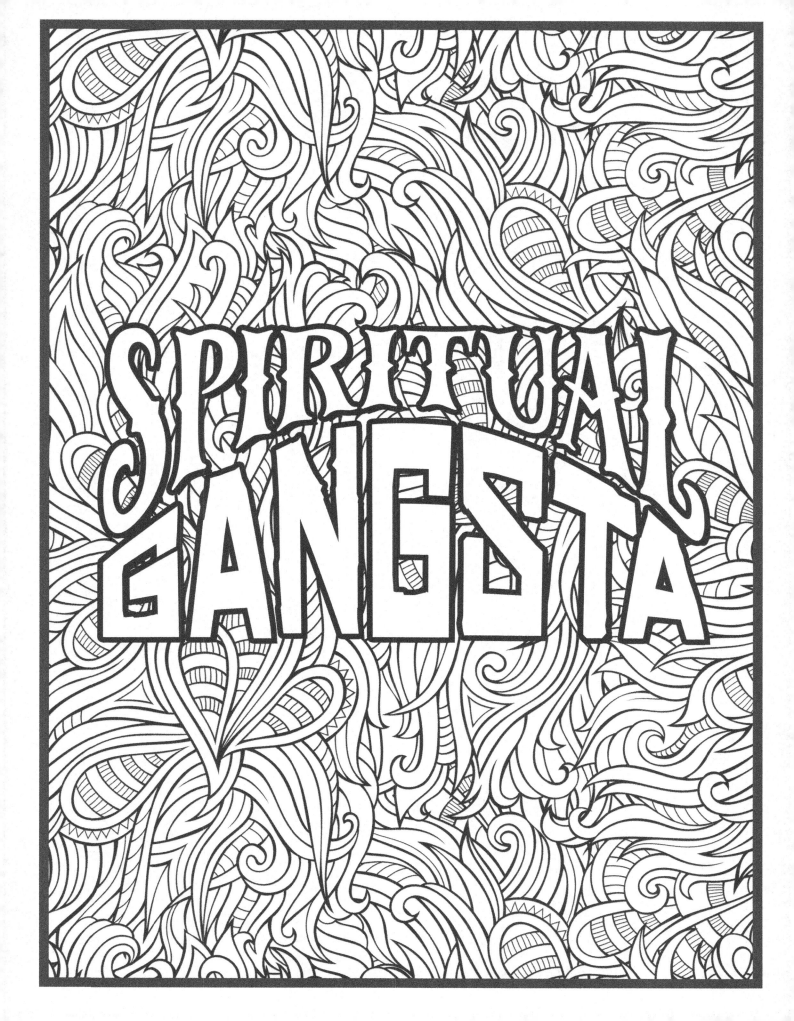

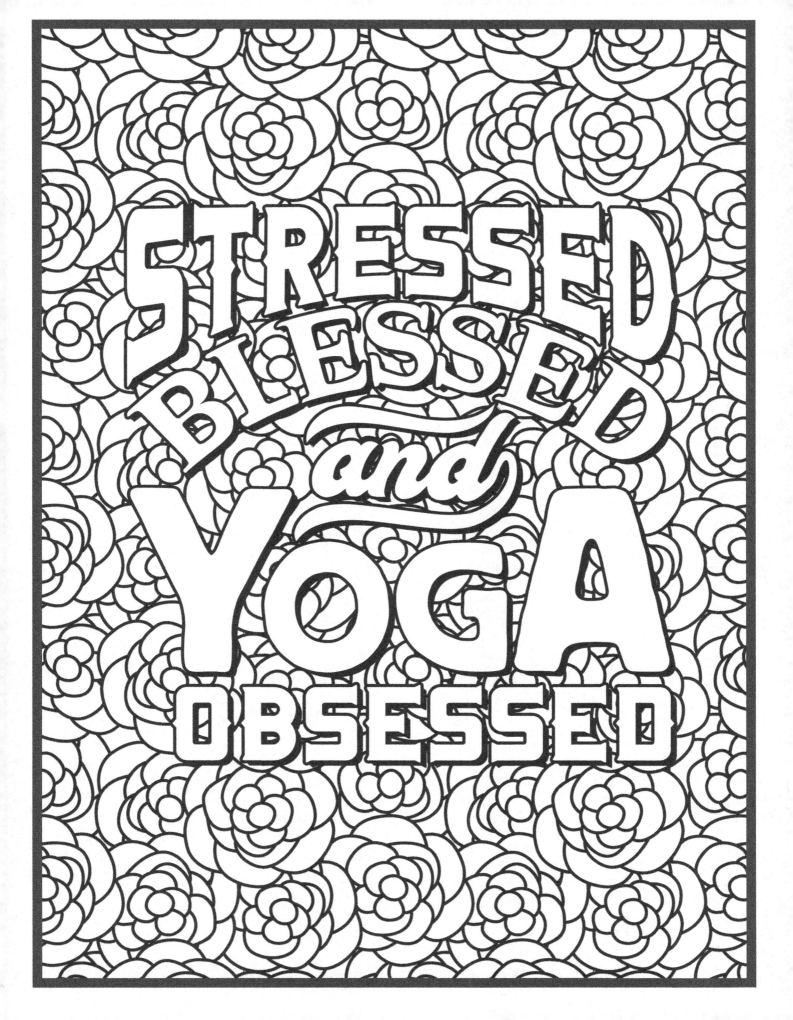

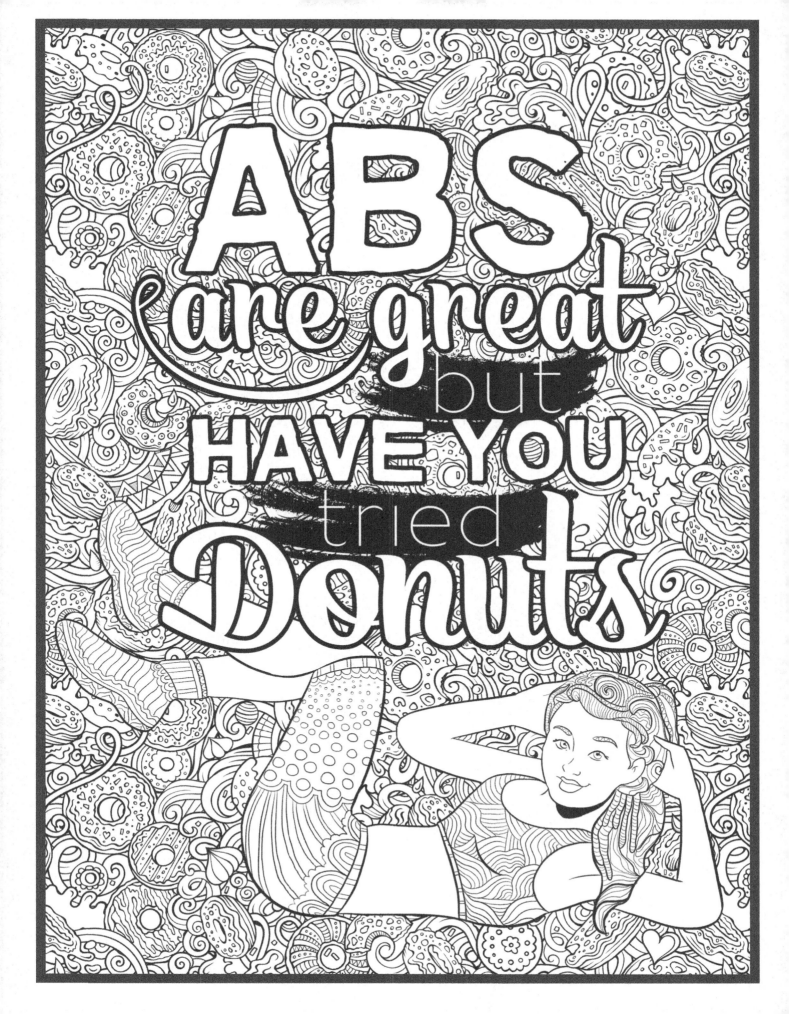

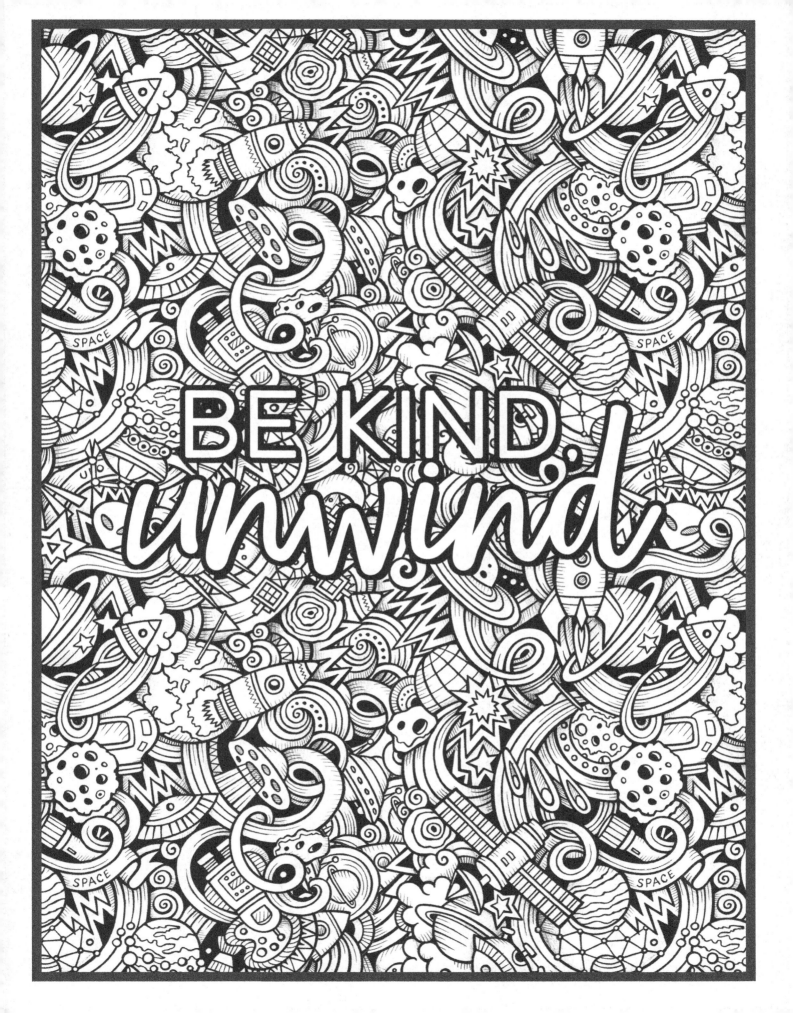

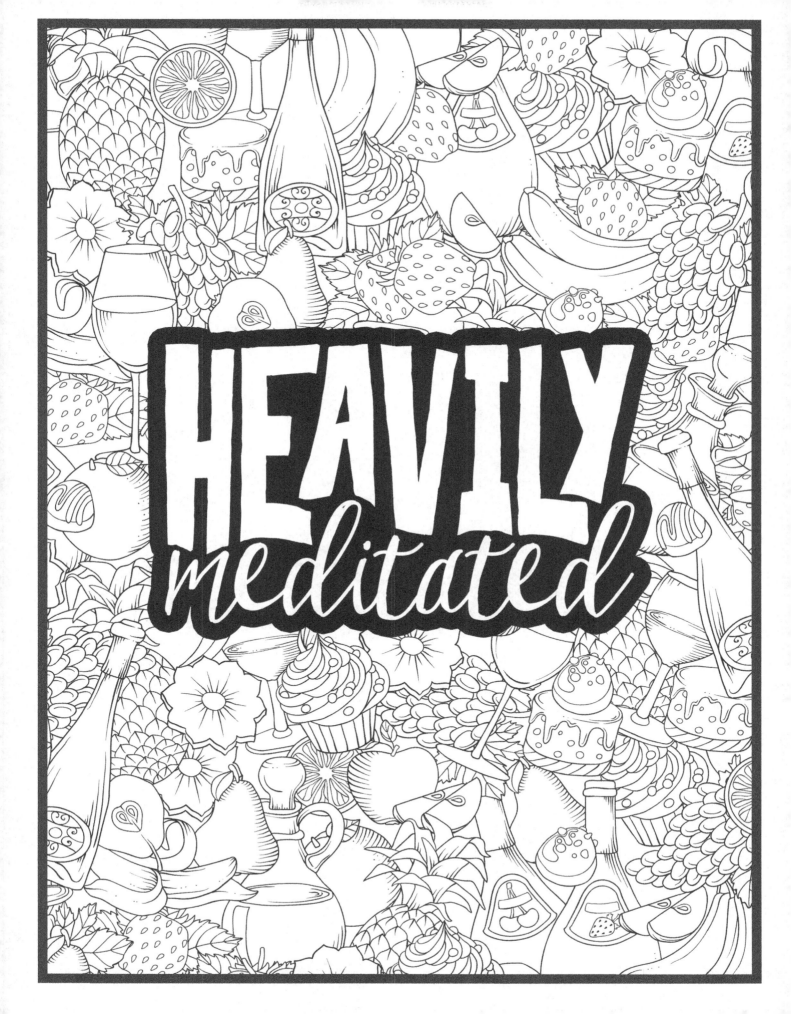

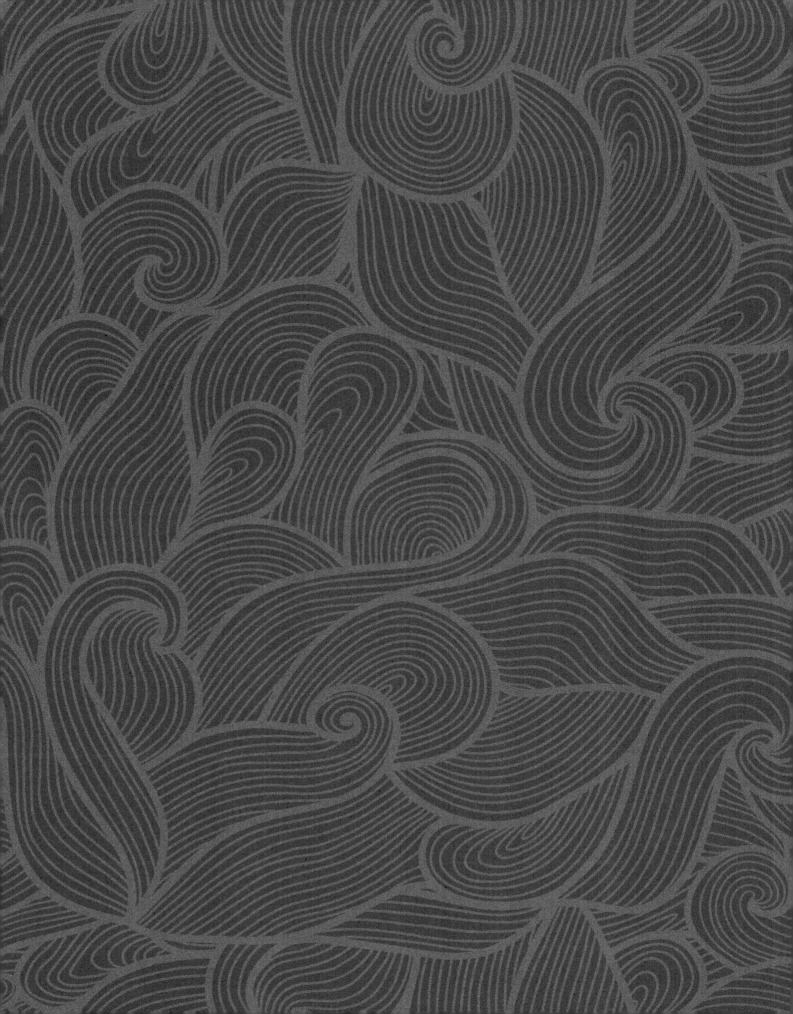

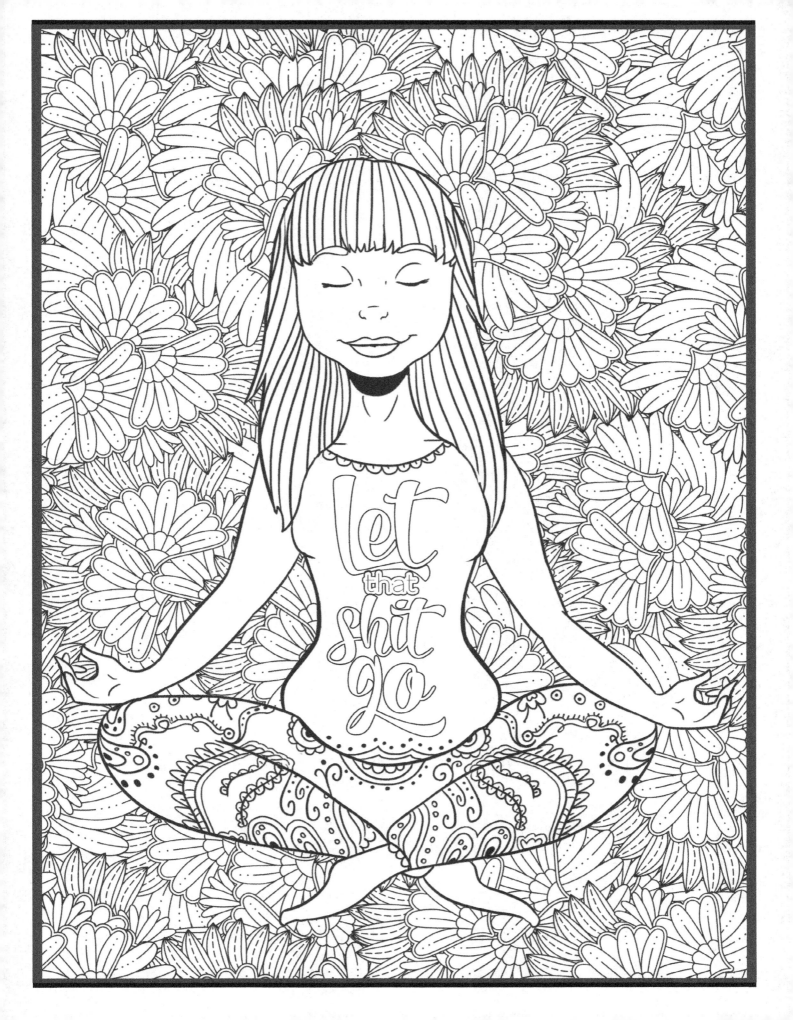

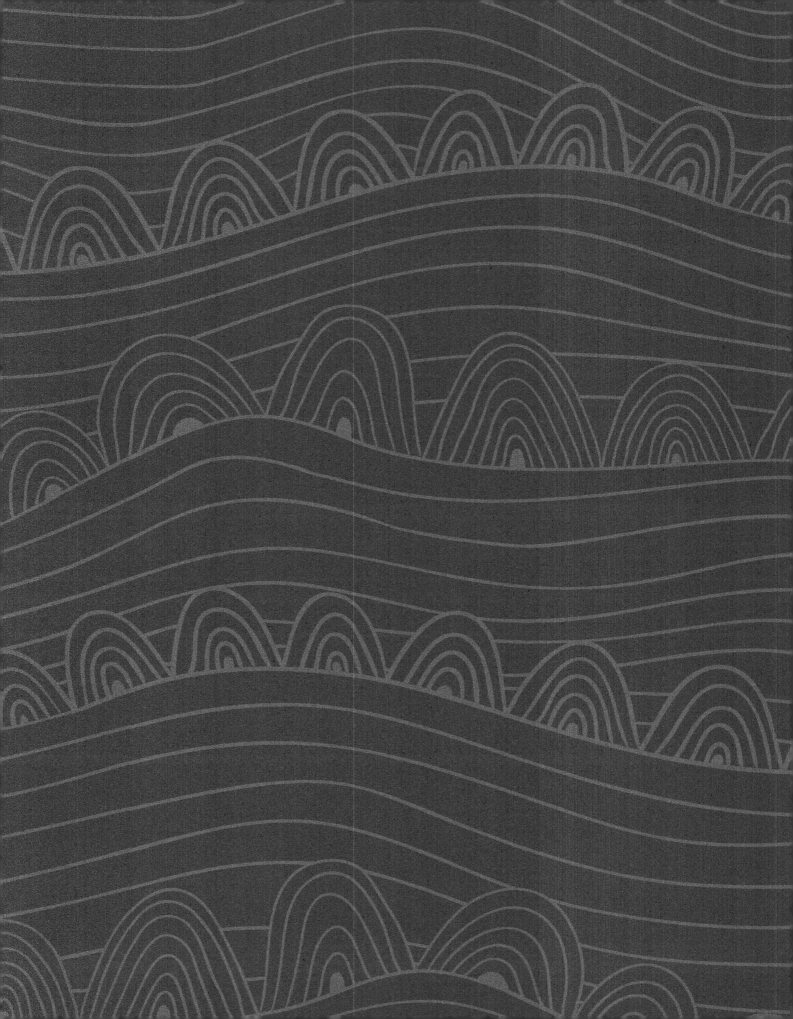

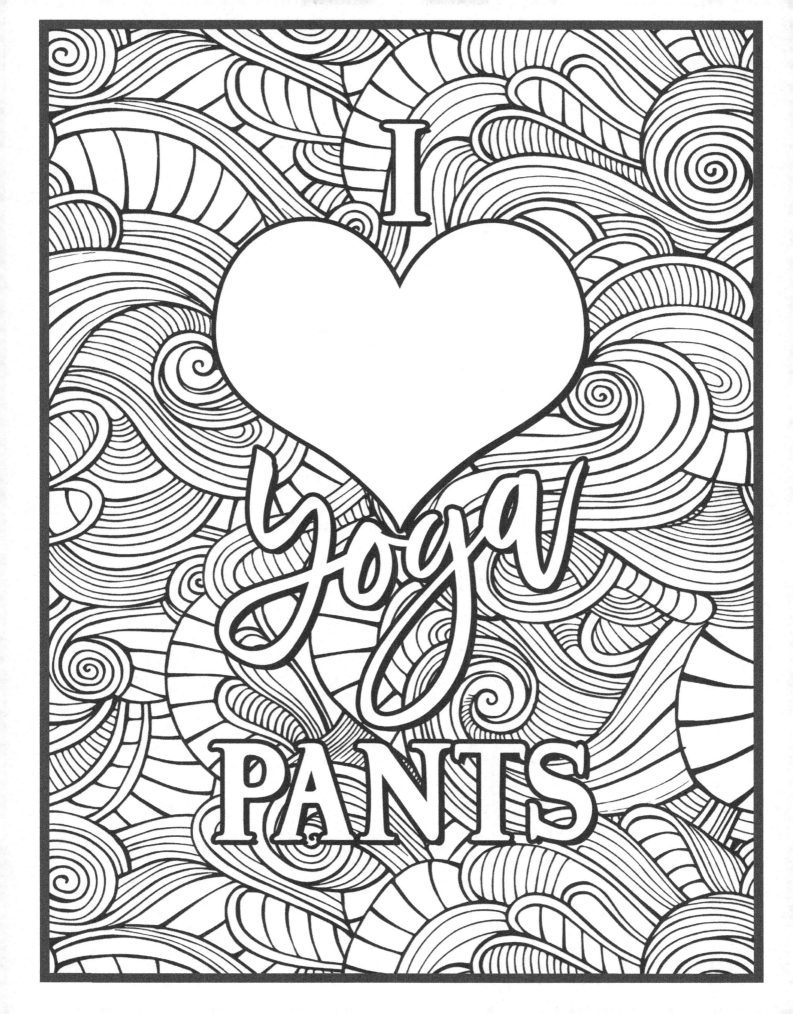

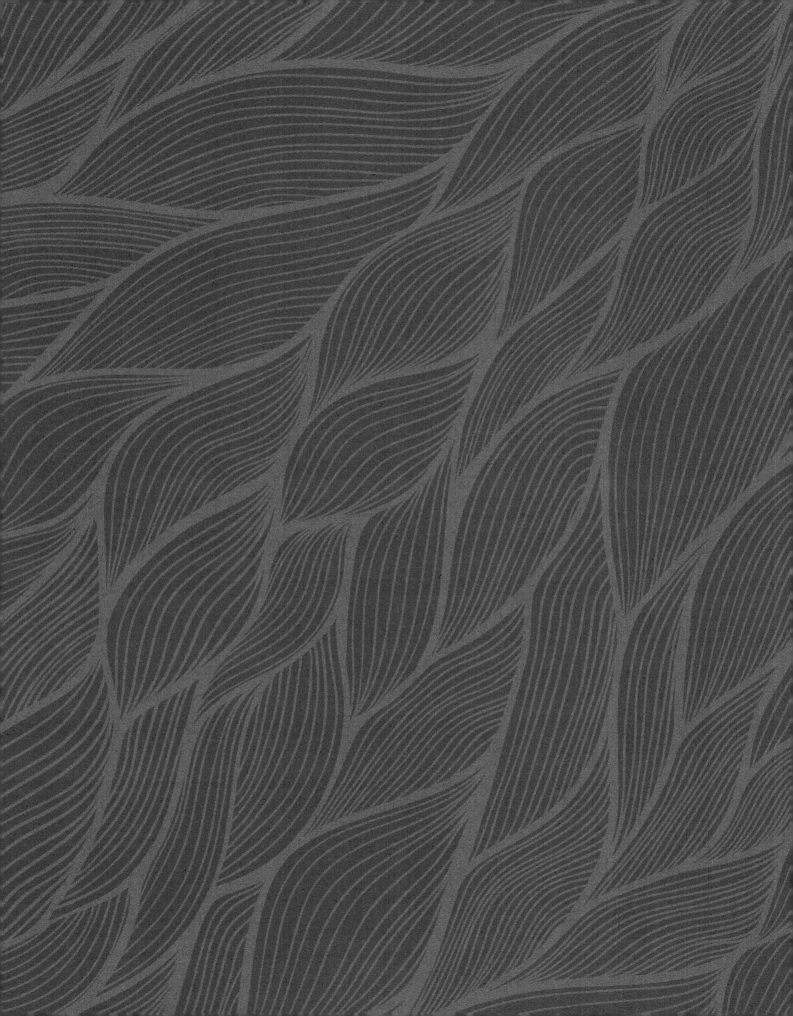

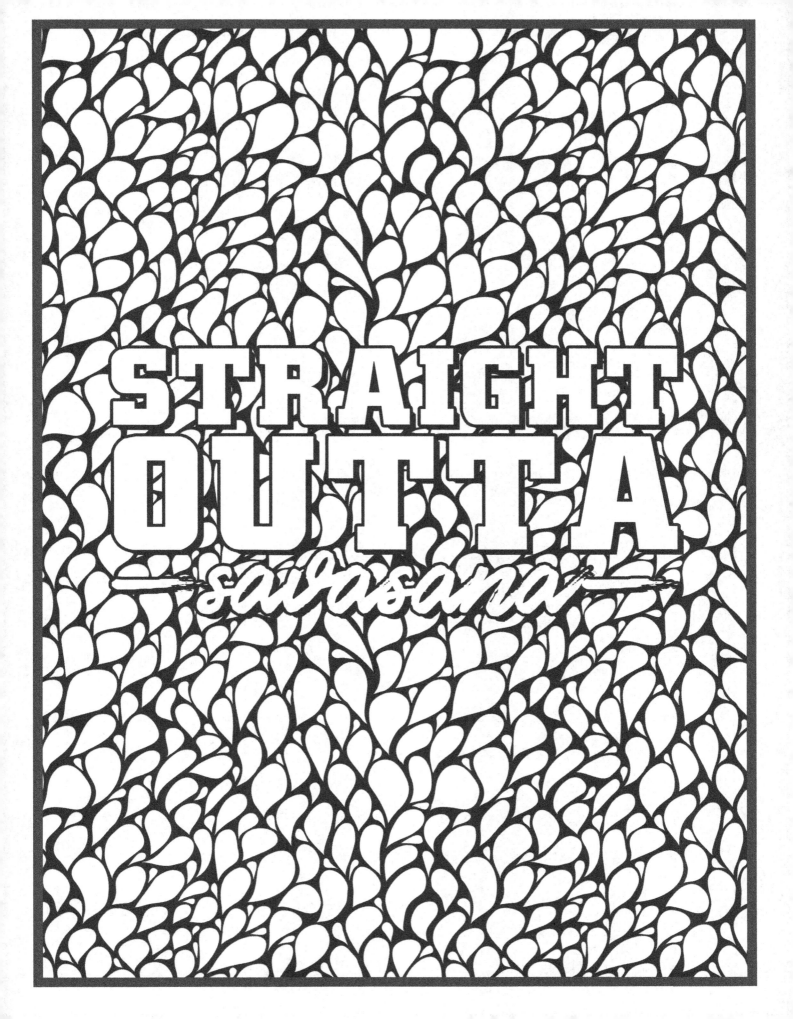

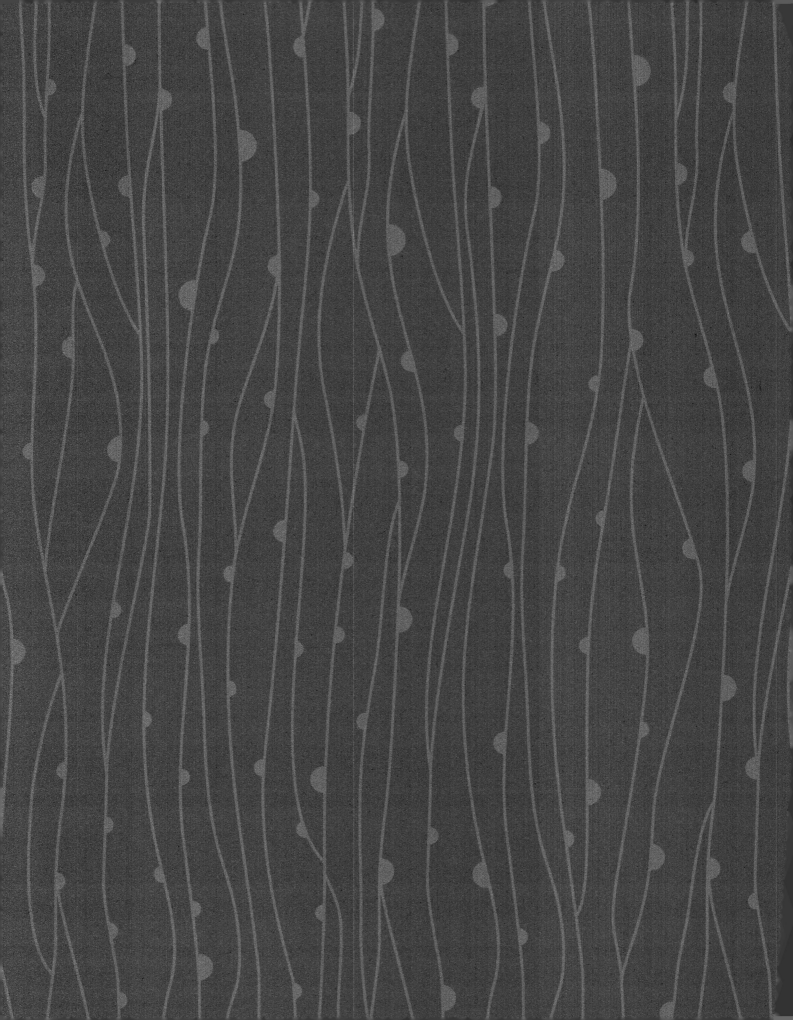

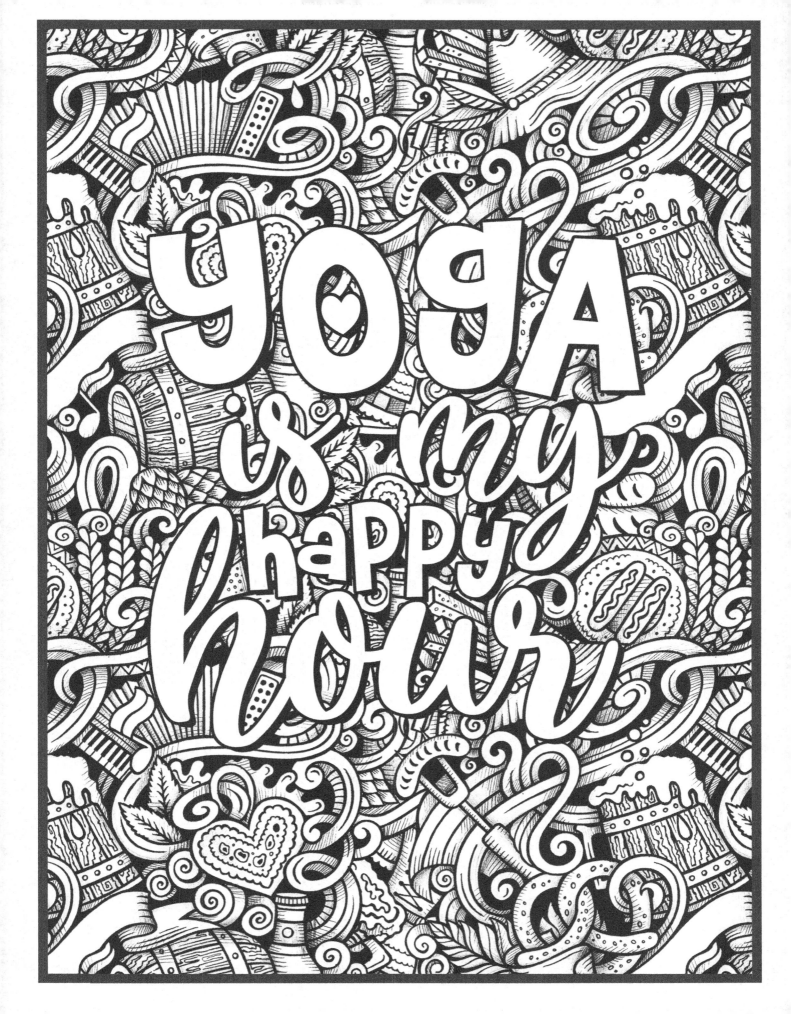

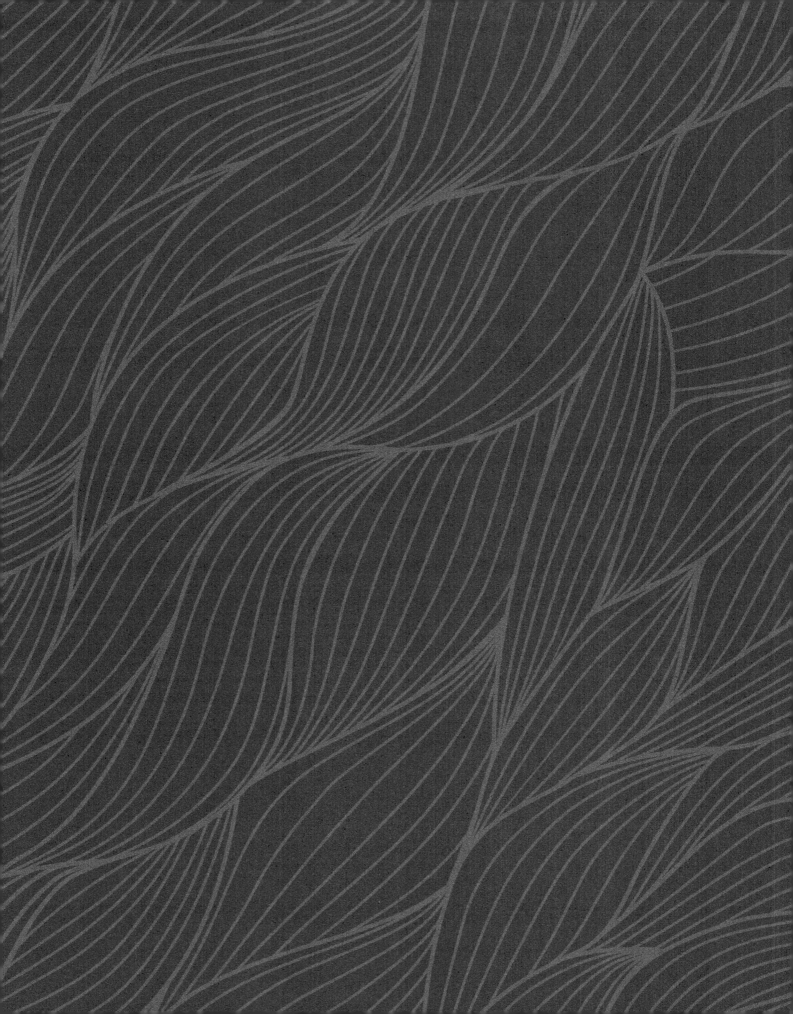

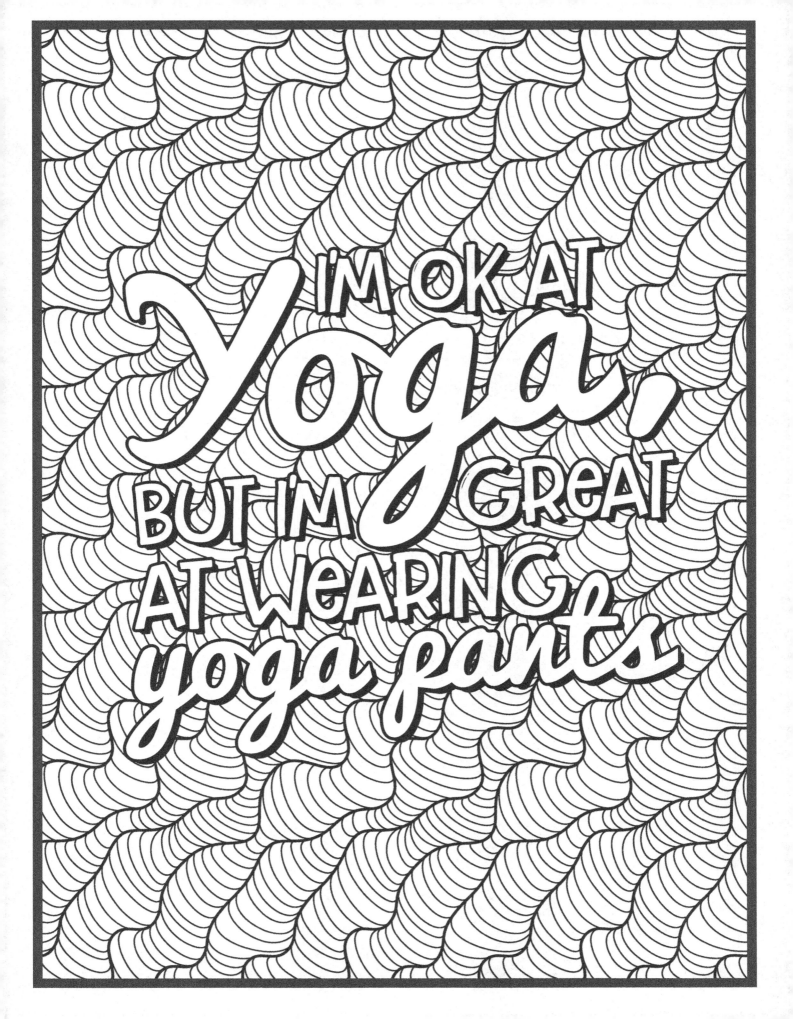

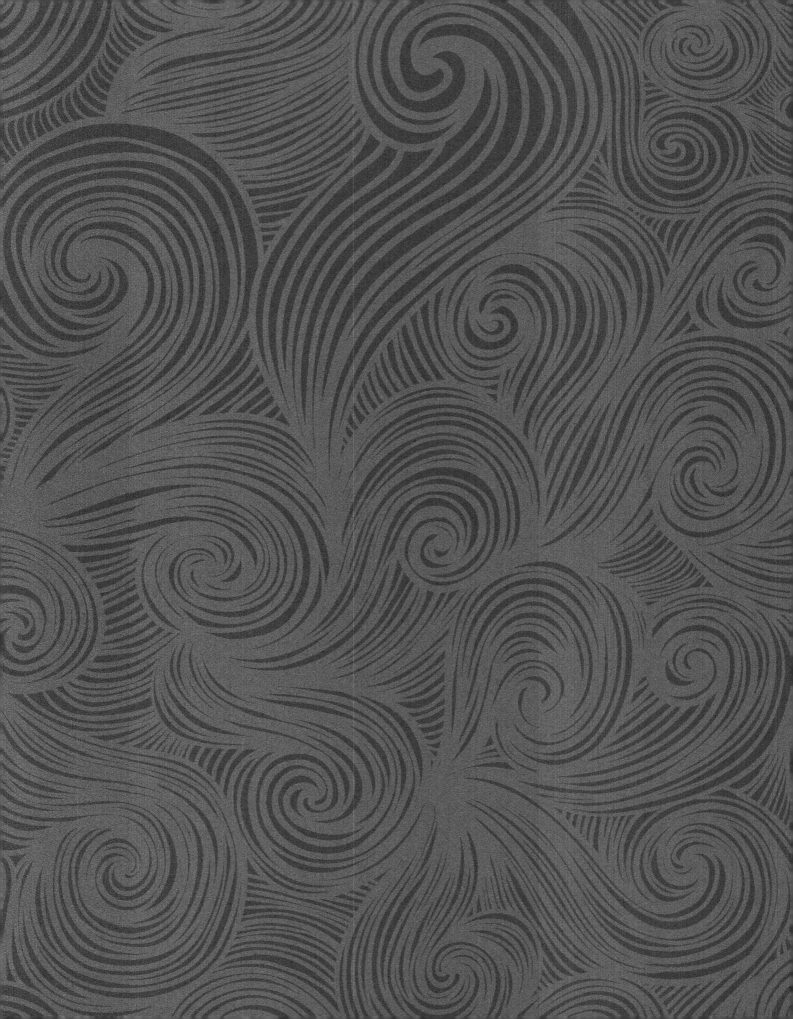

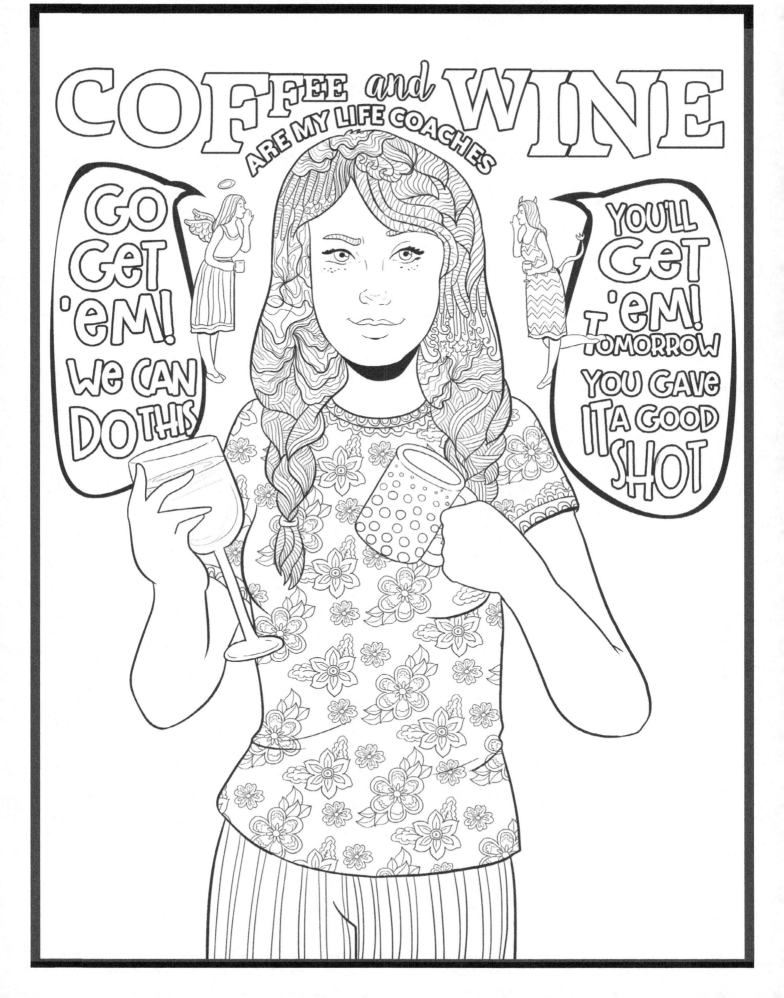

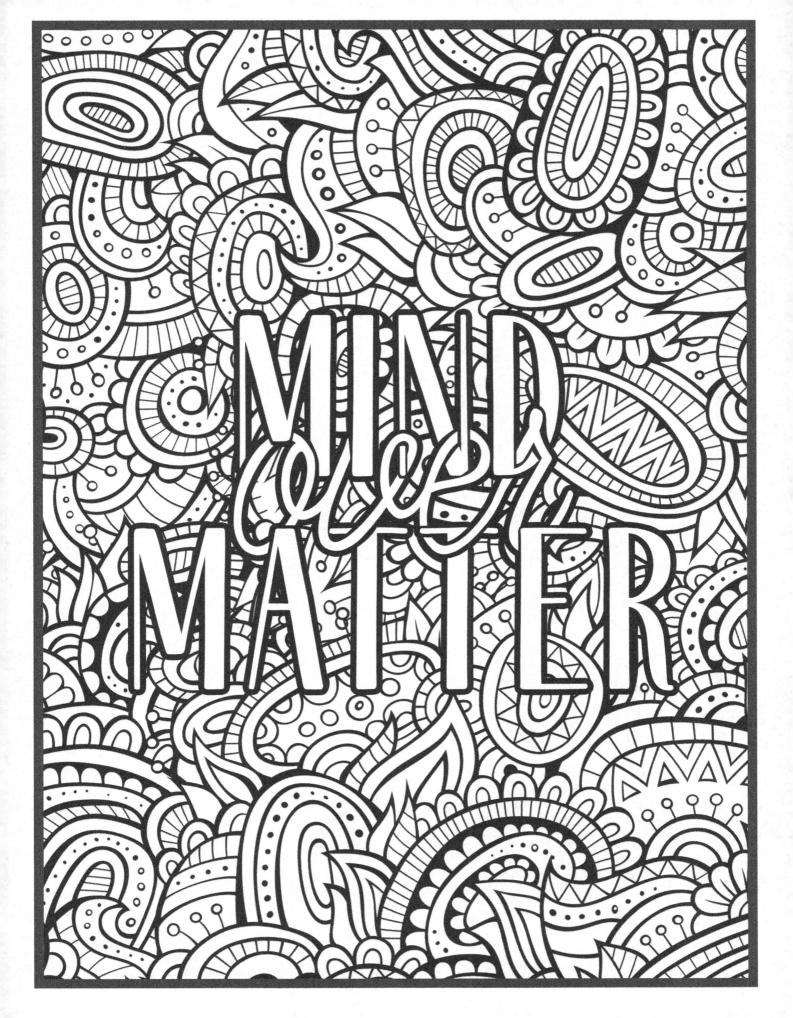

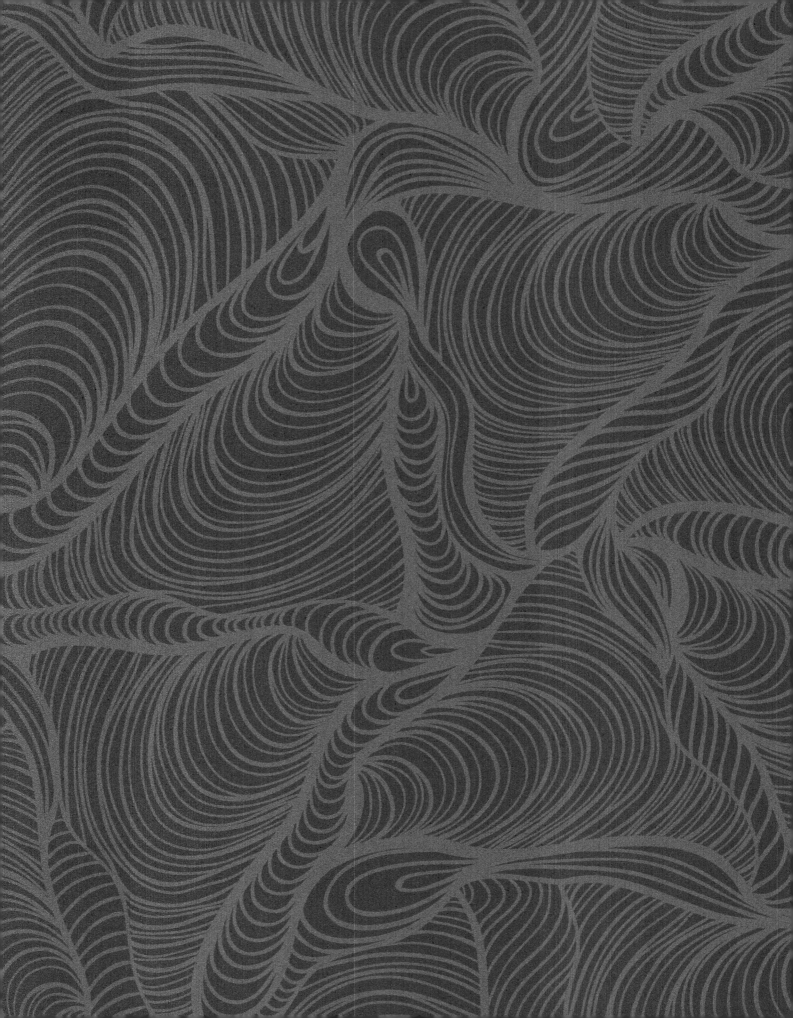

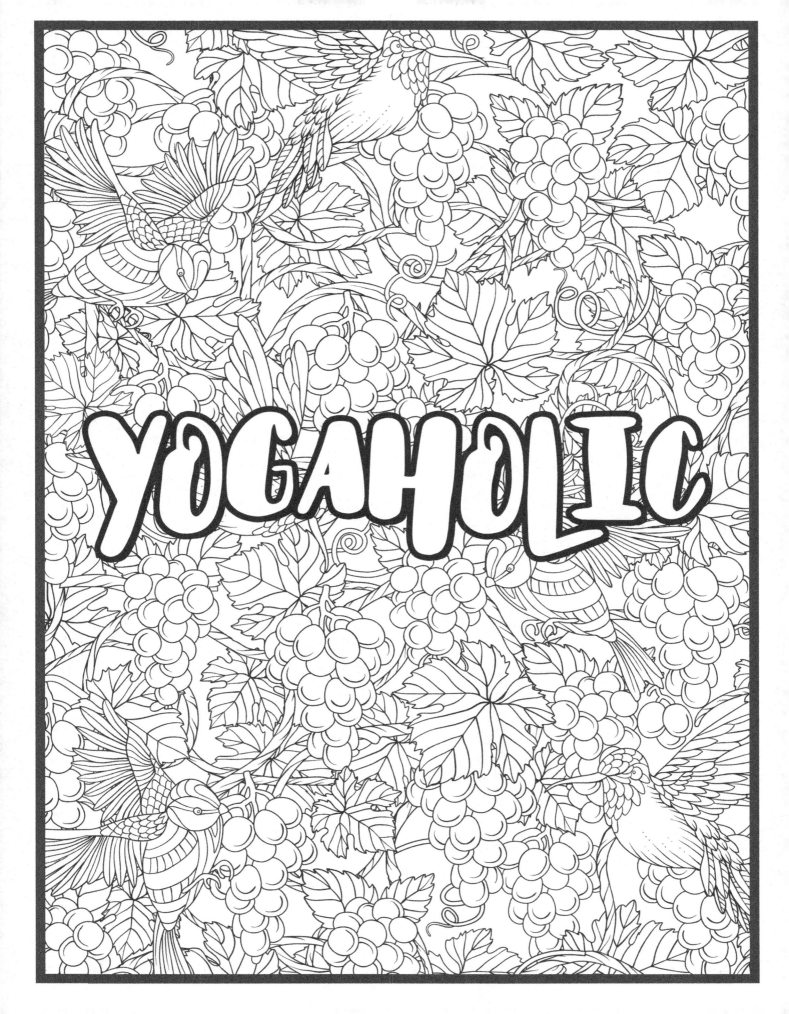

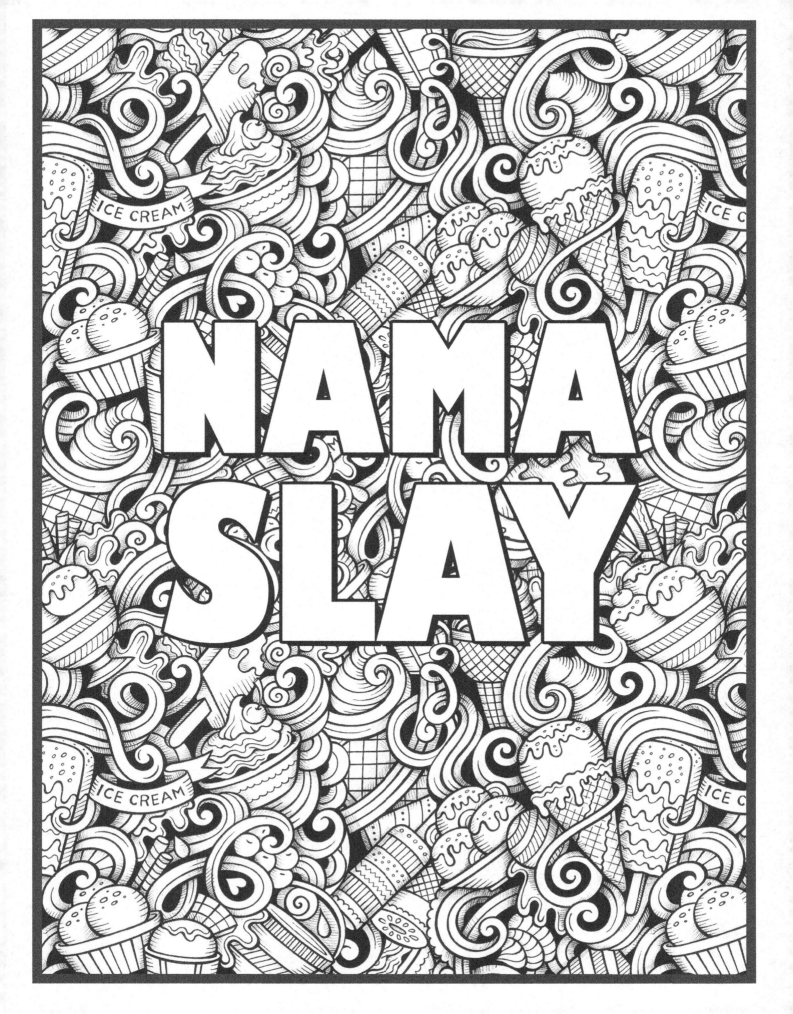

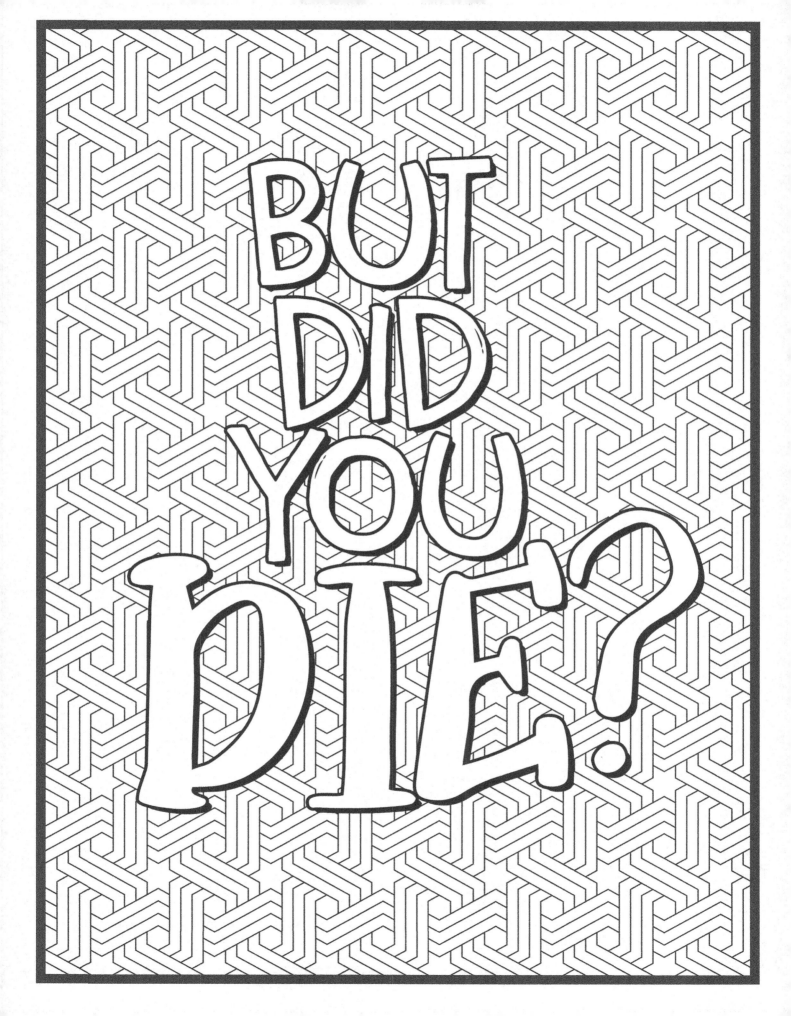

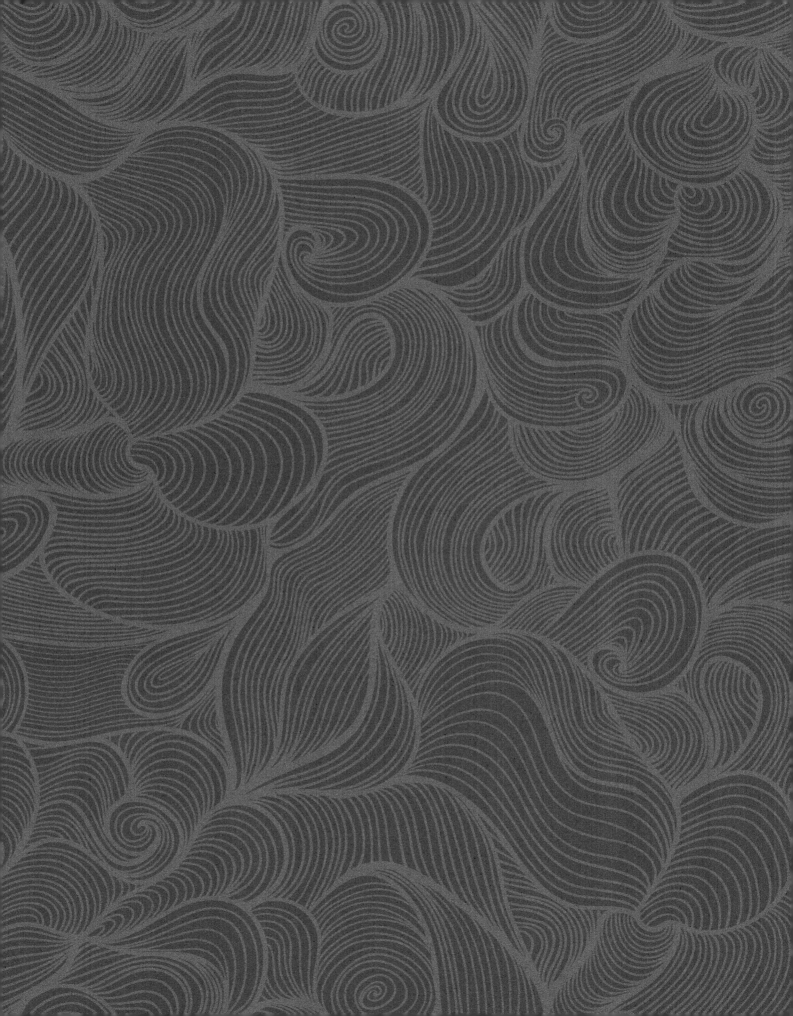

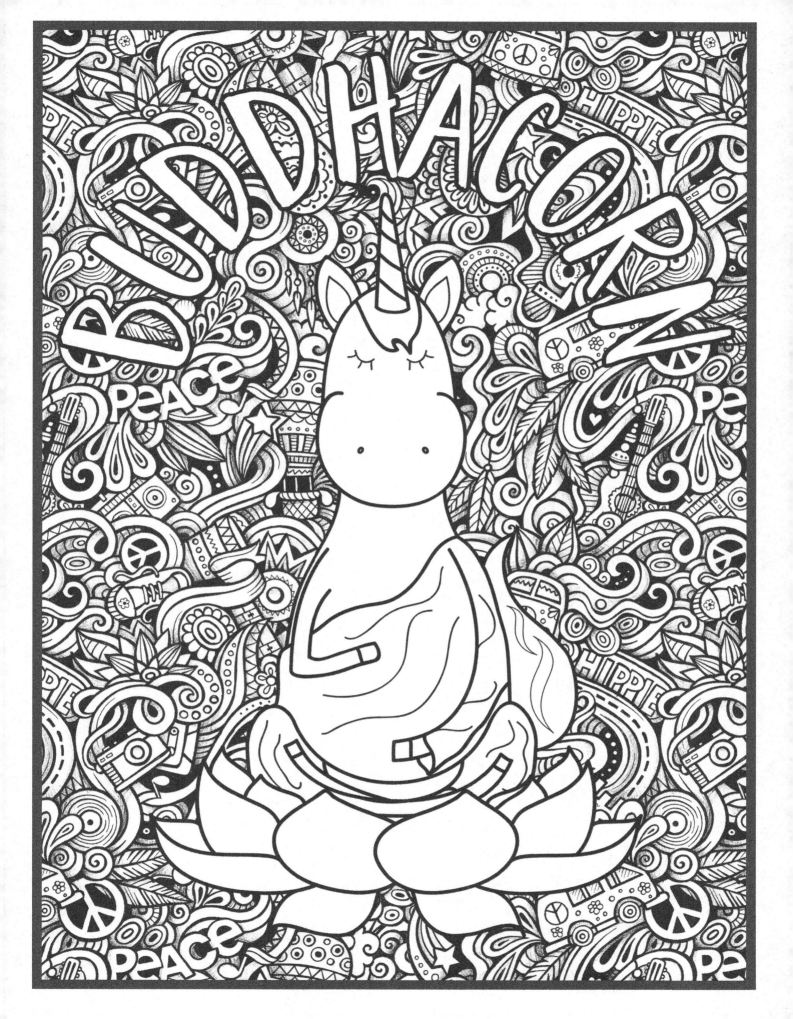

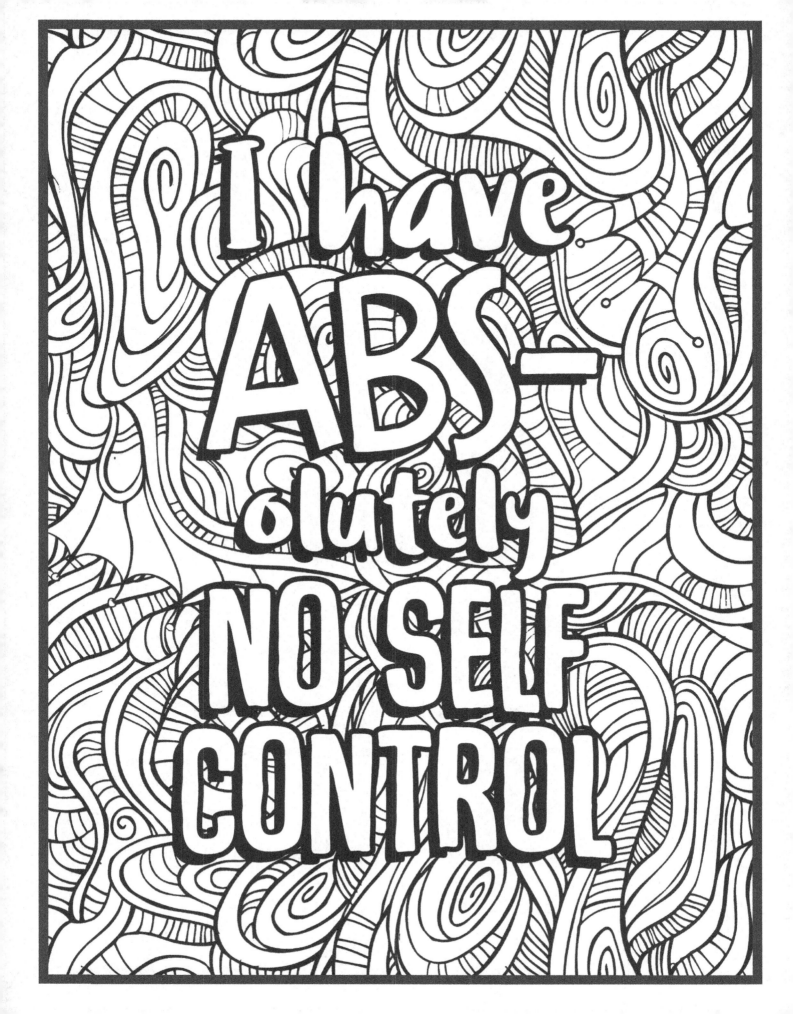

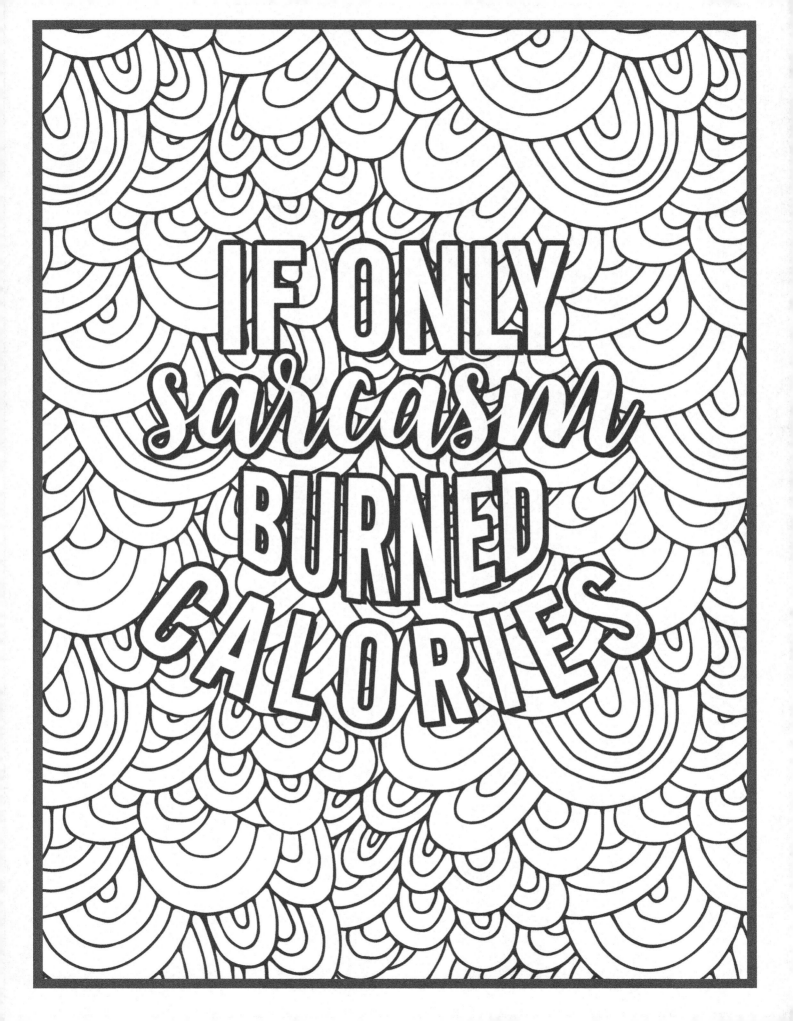

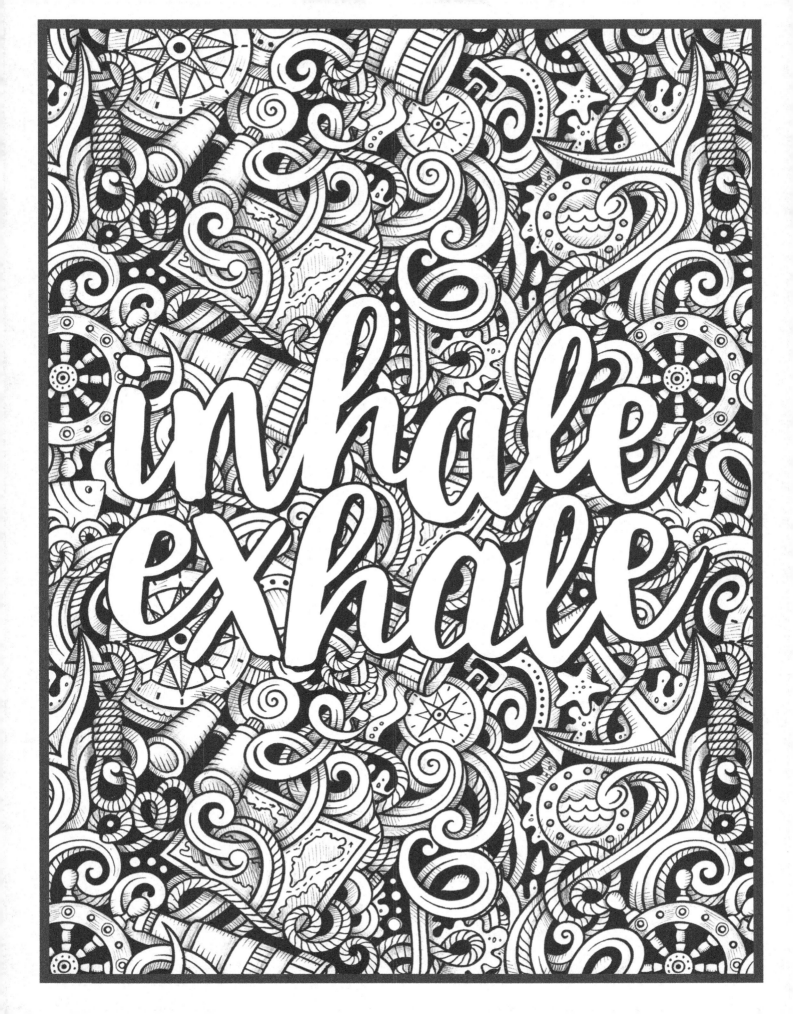

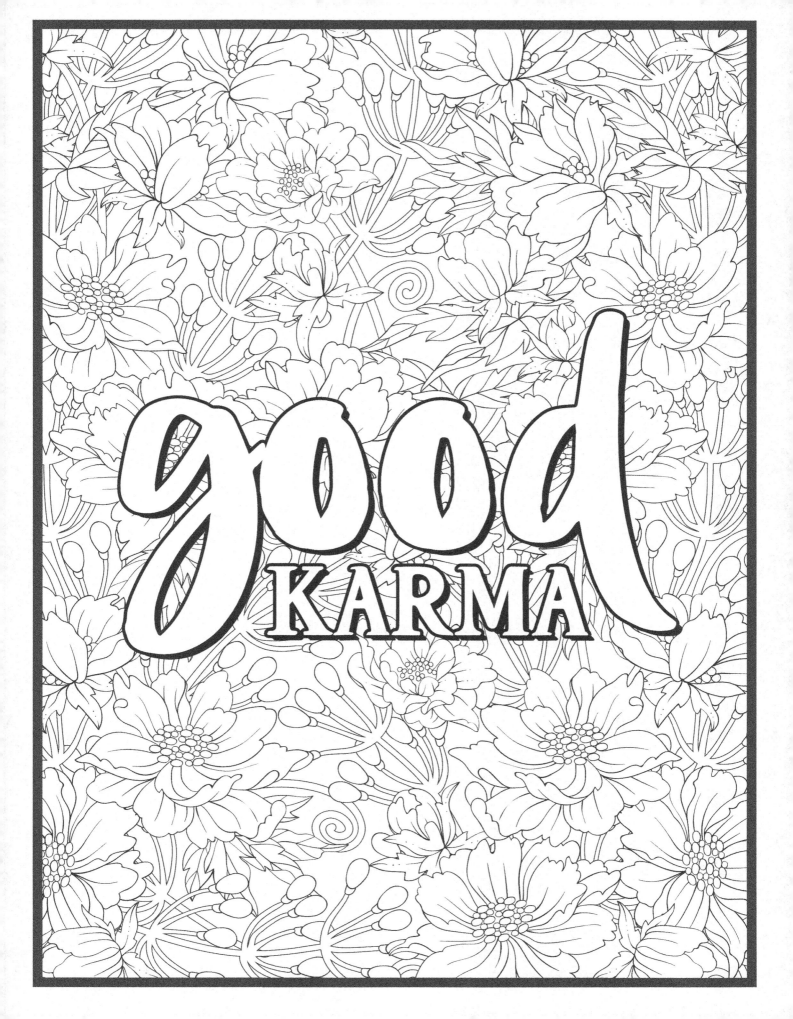

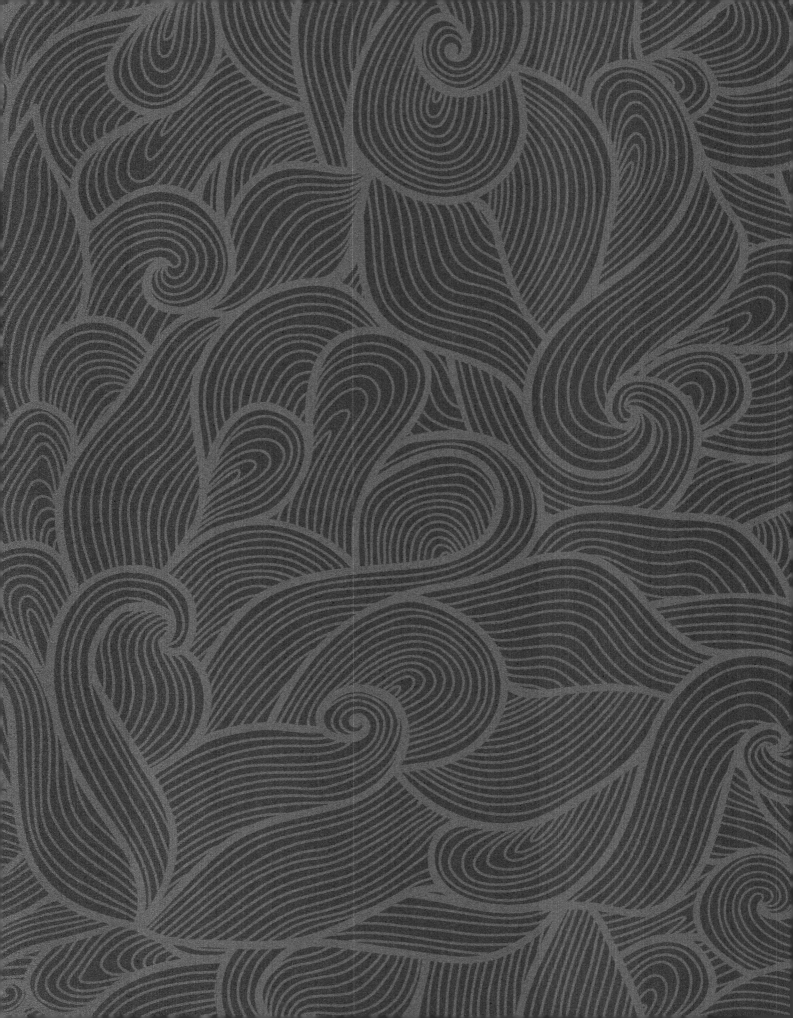

I ENJOY 1 GLASS OF WINE each night FOR THE HEALTH BENEFITS. & THE other GLASSES ARE FOR WITTY comebacks & flawless DANCE MOVES!

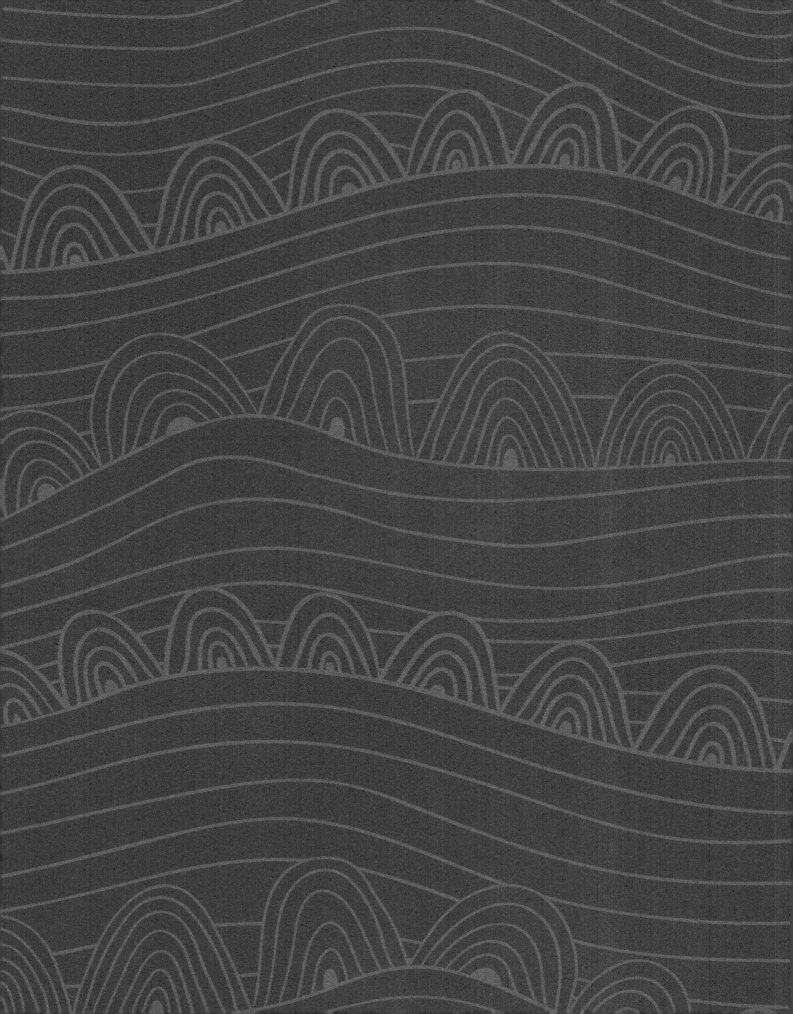

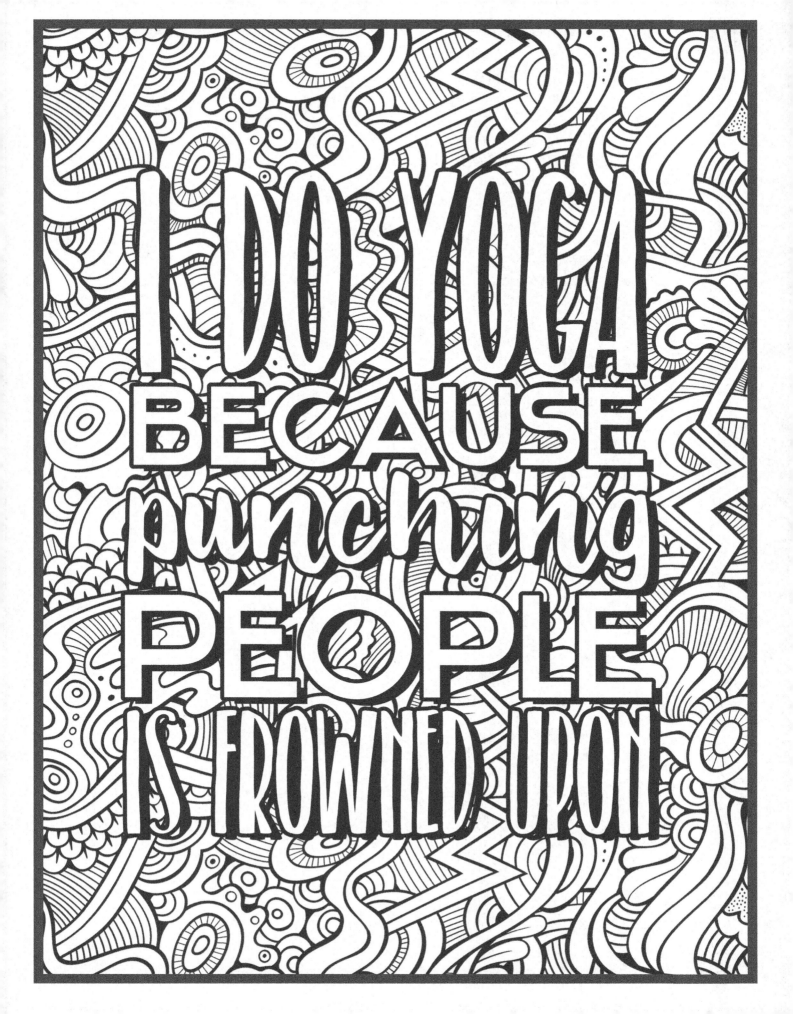

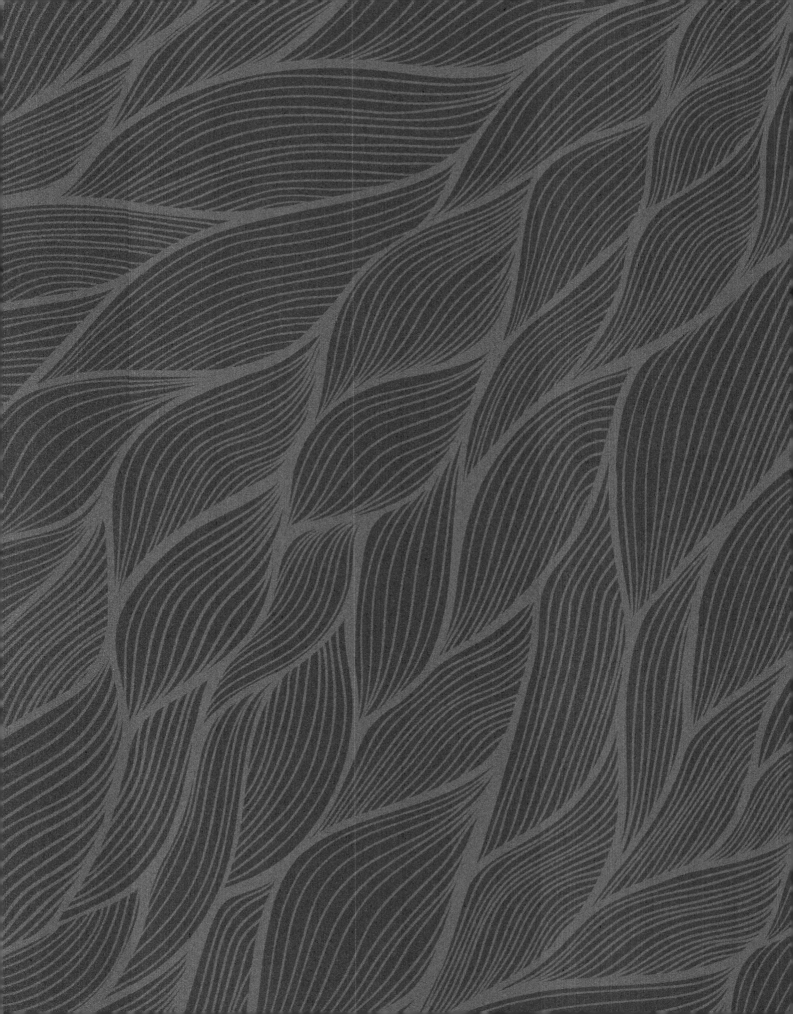

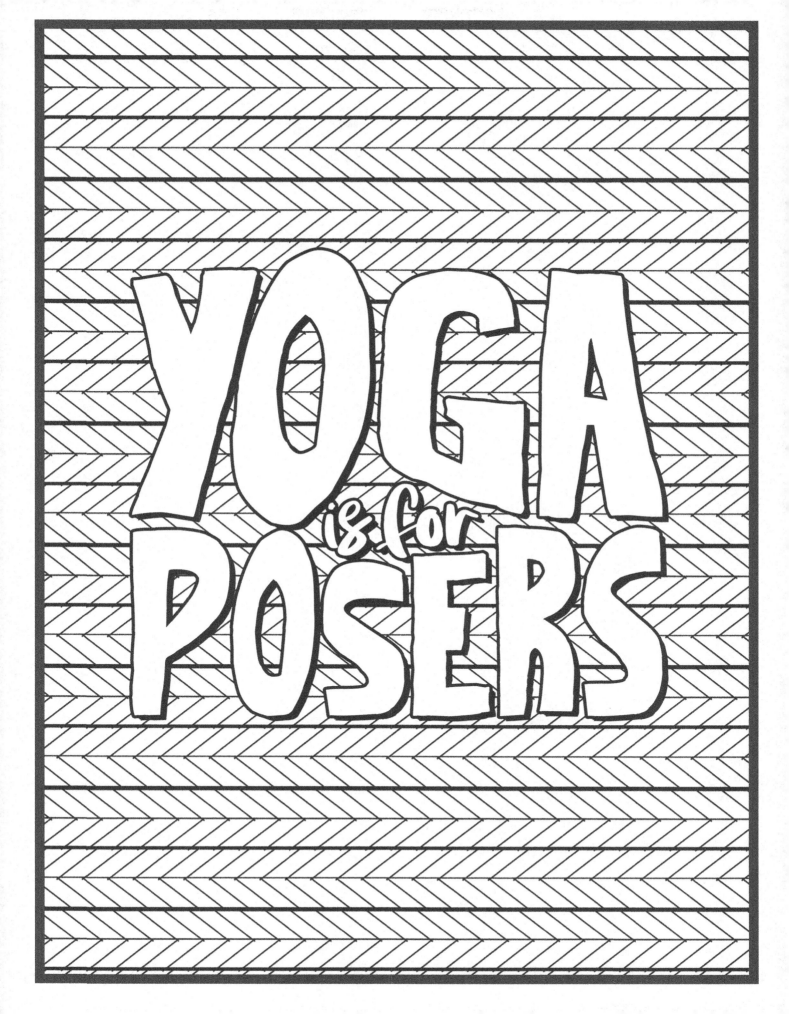

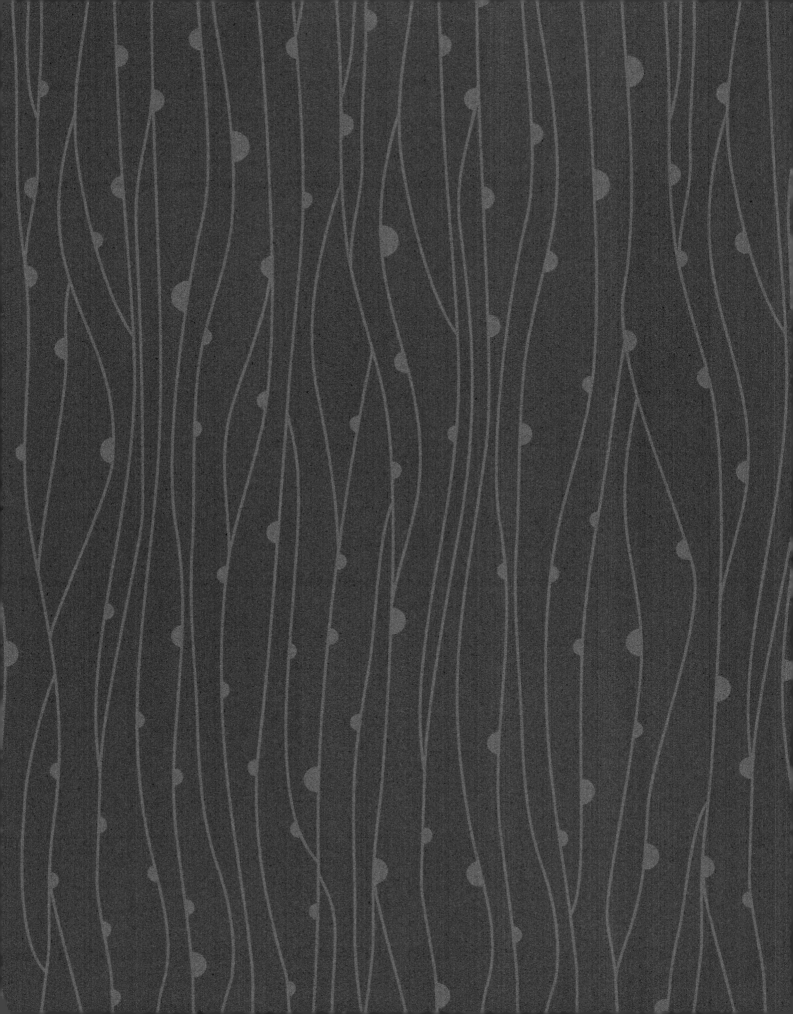

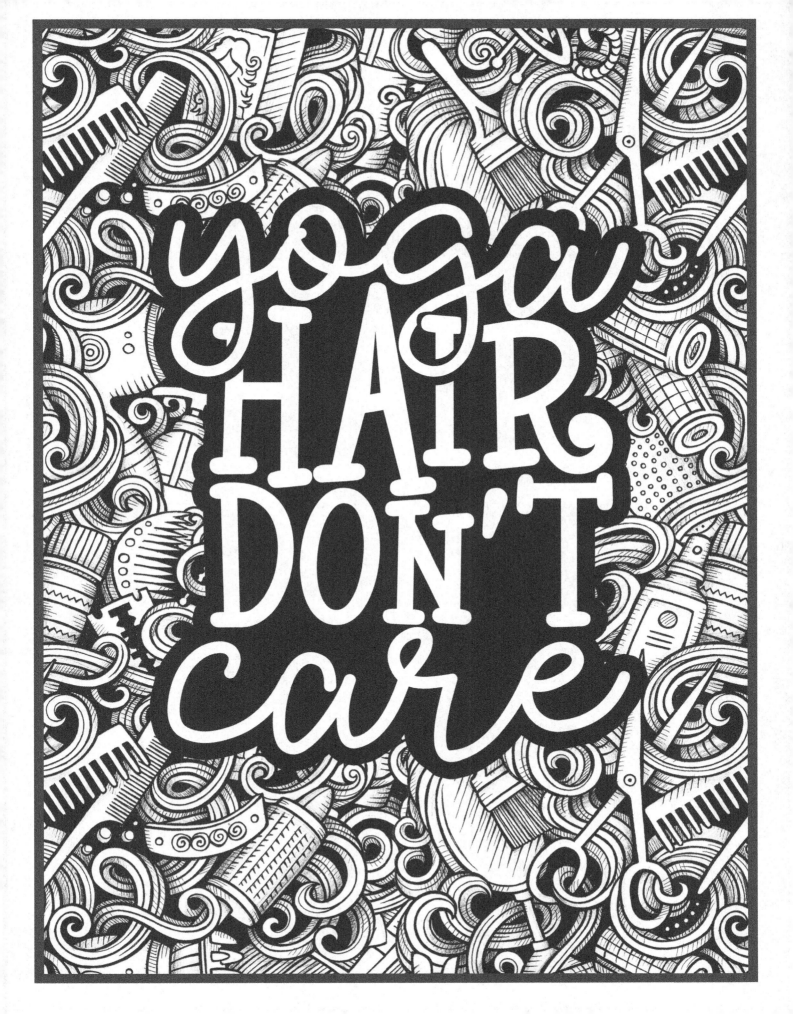

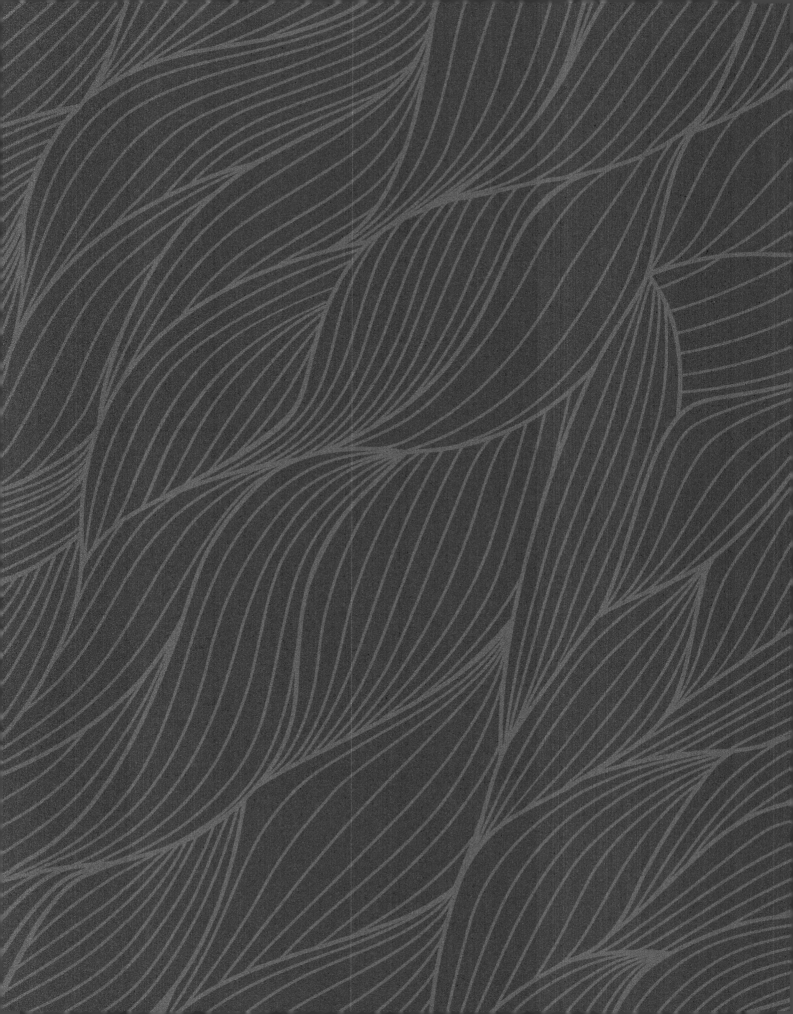

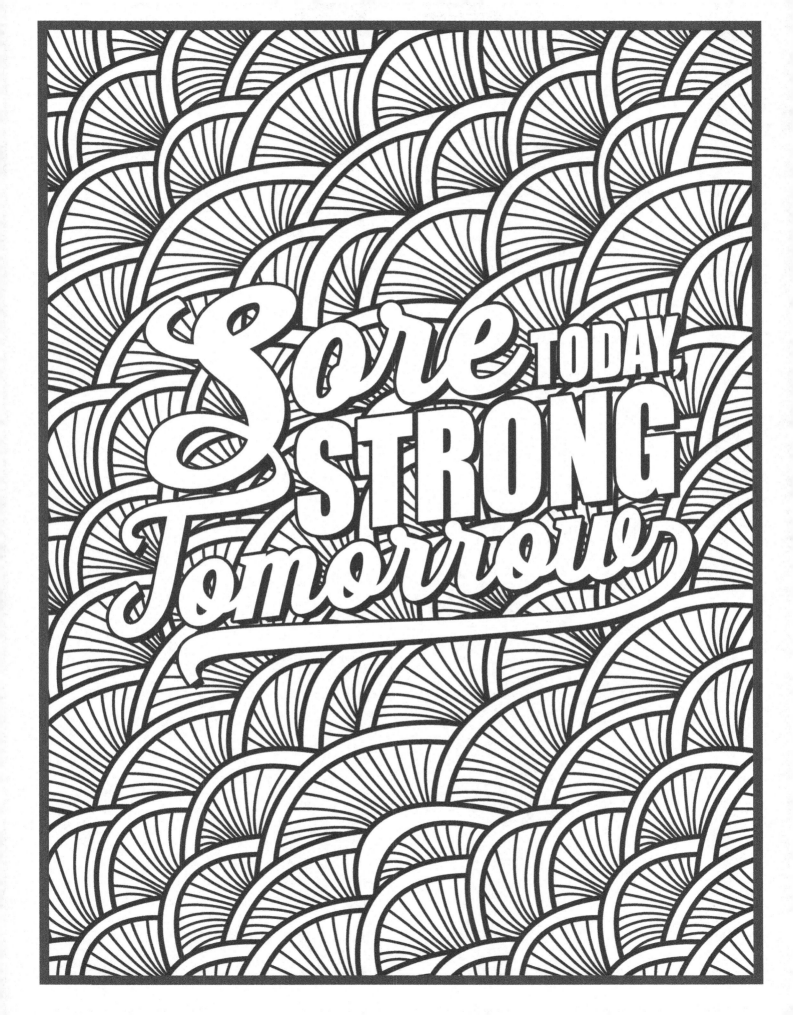

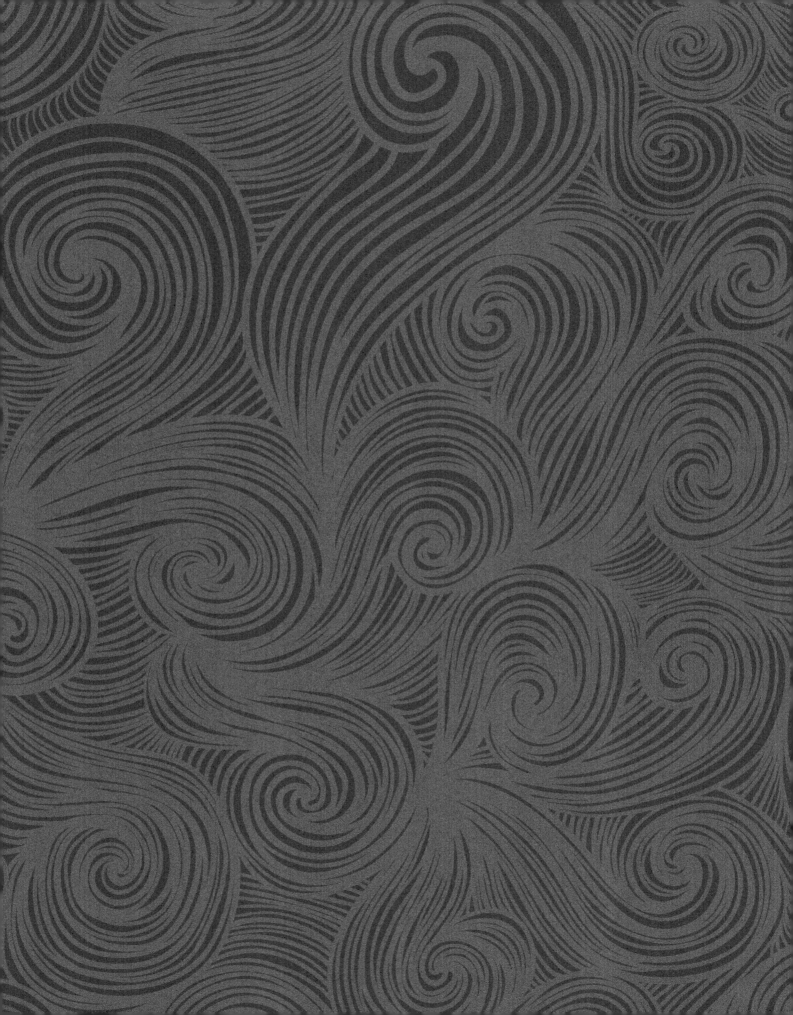

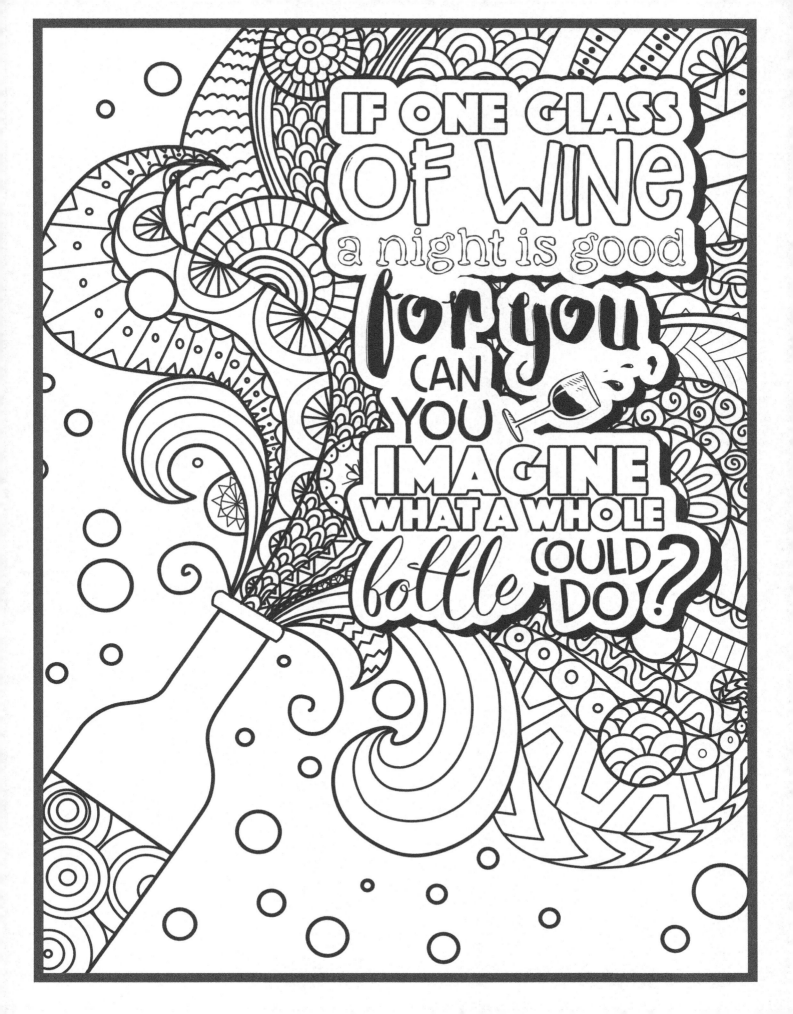

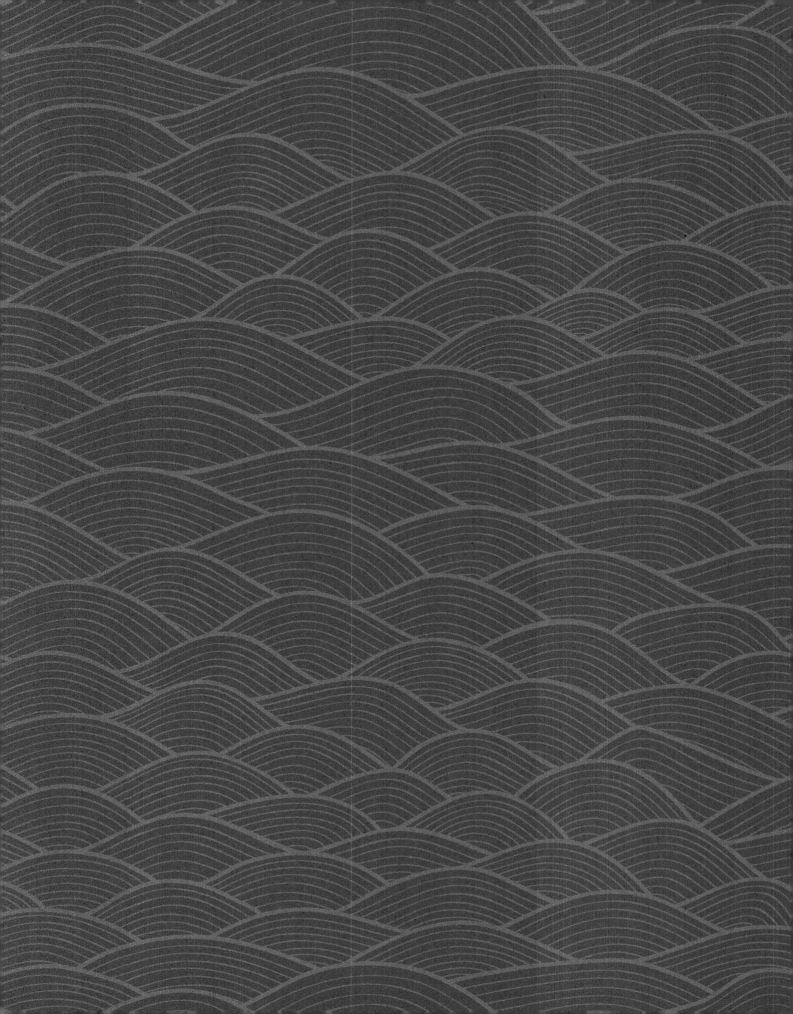

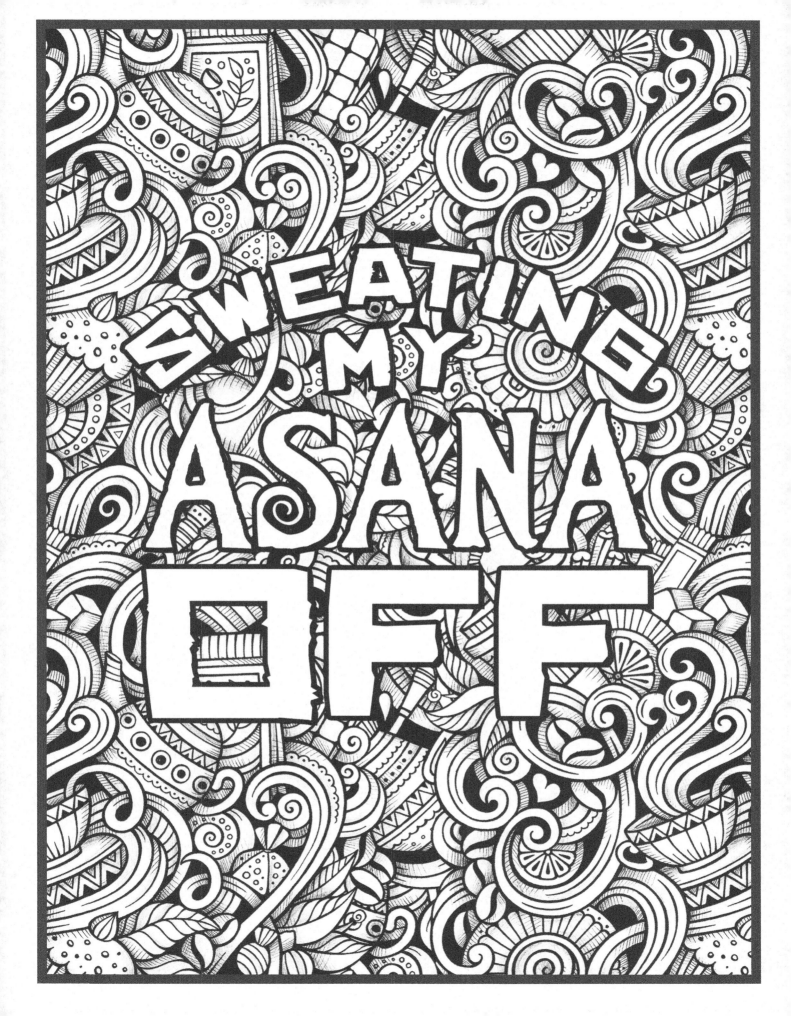

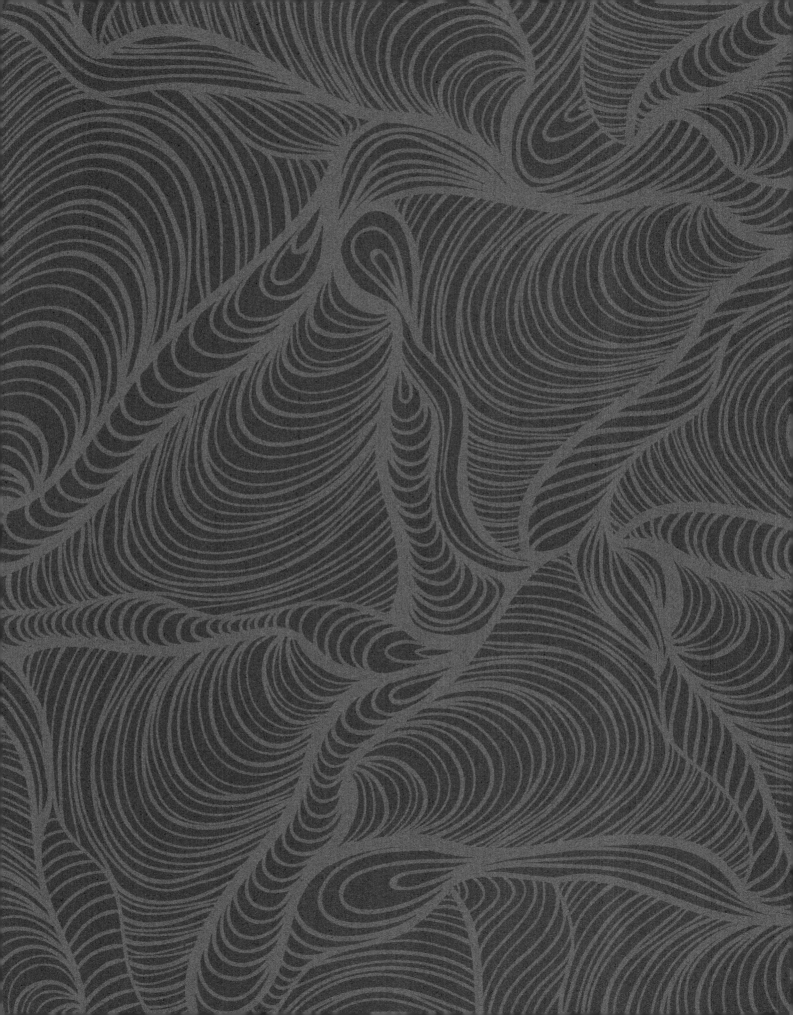

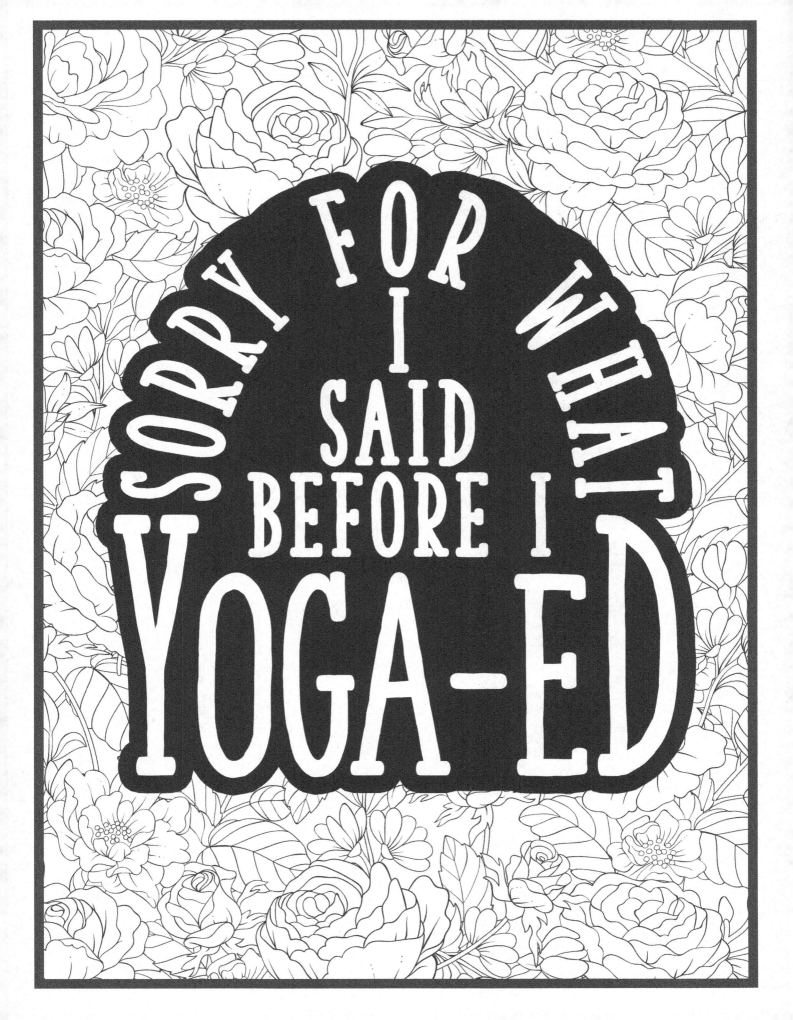

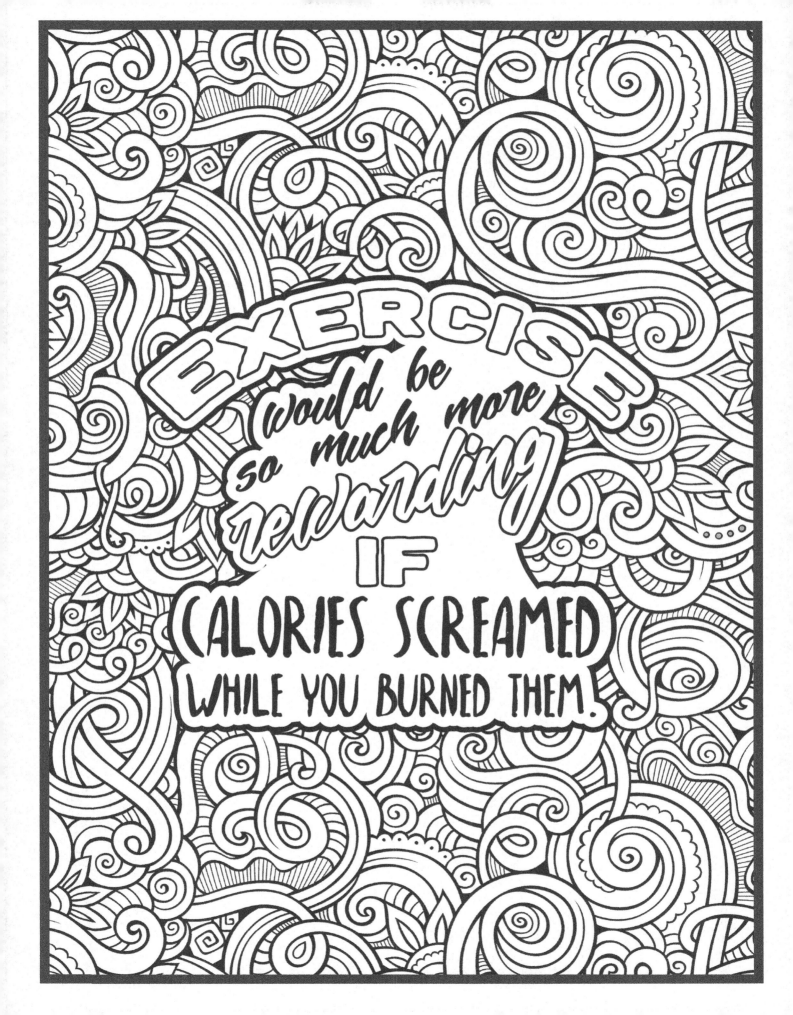

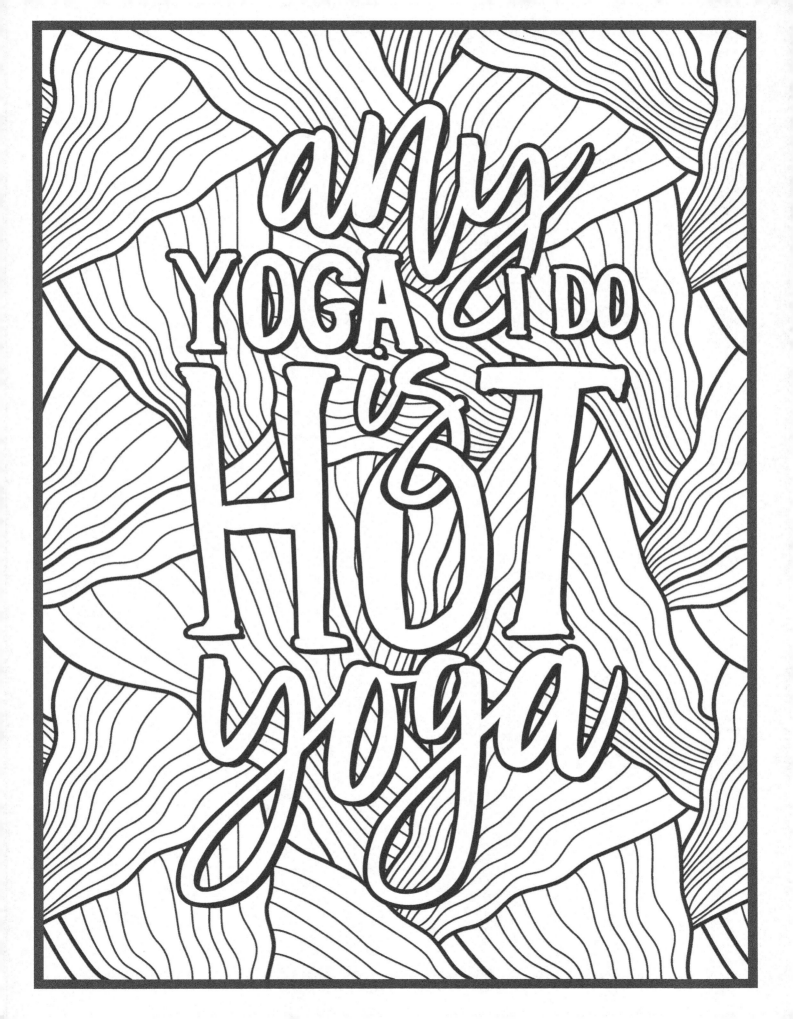

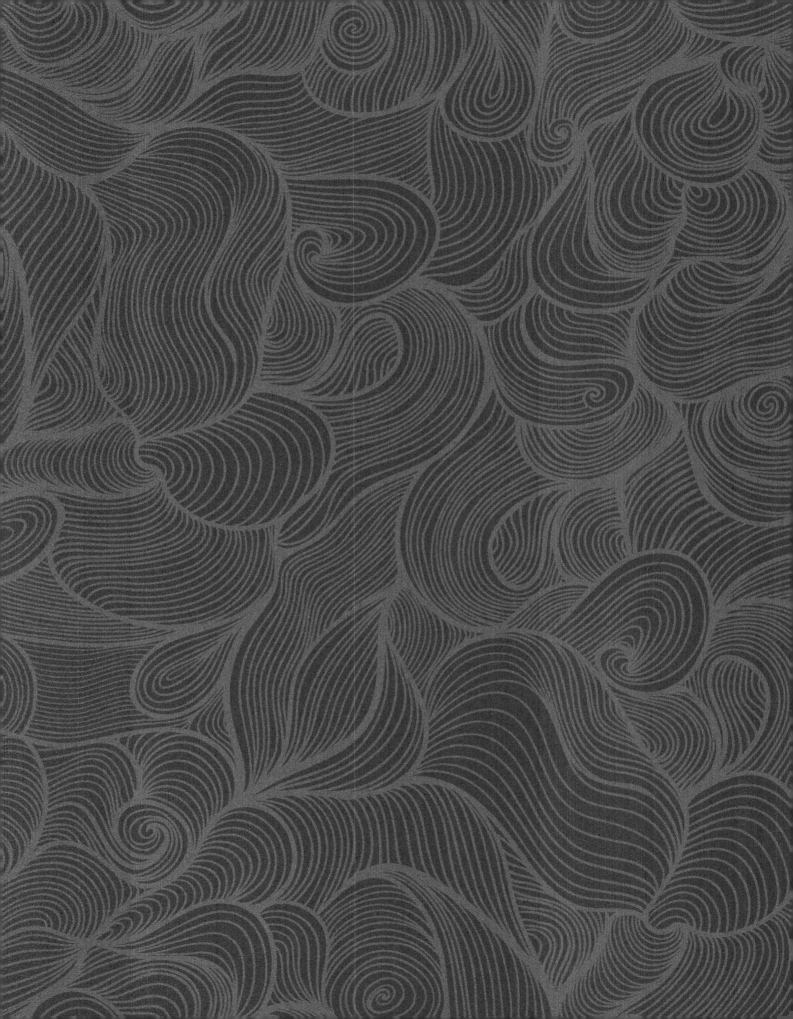

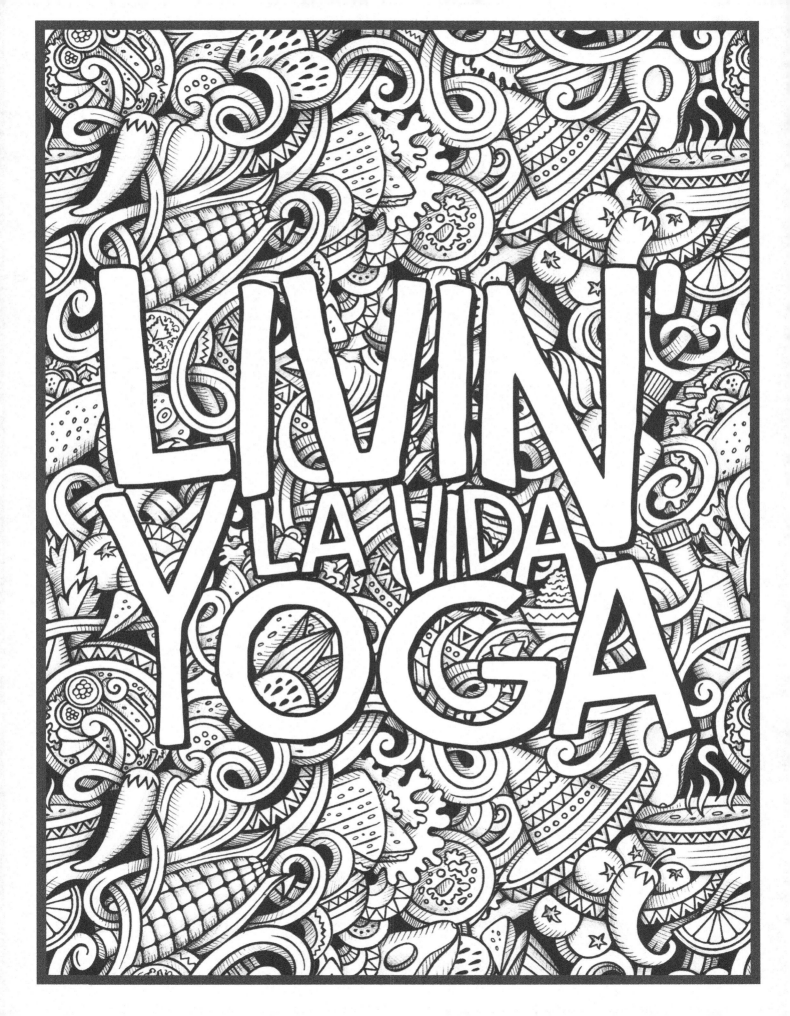

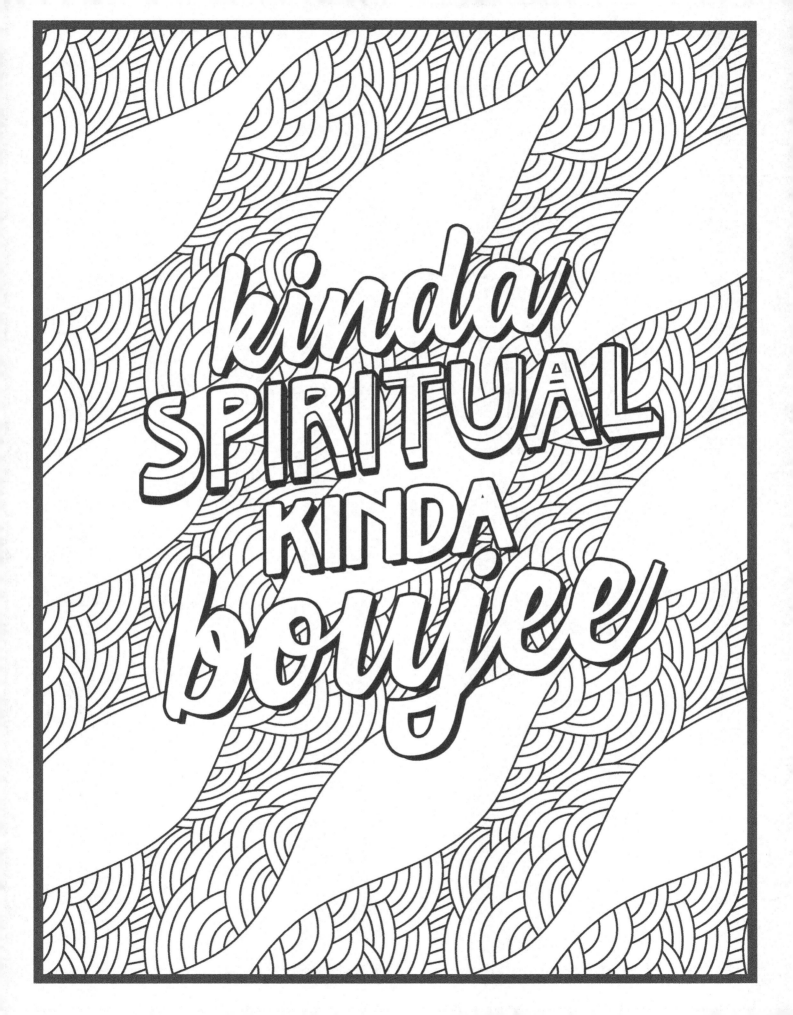

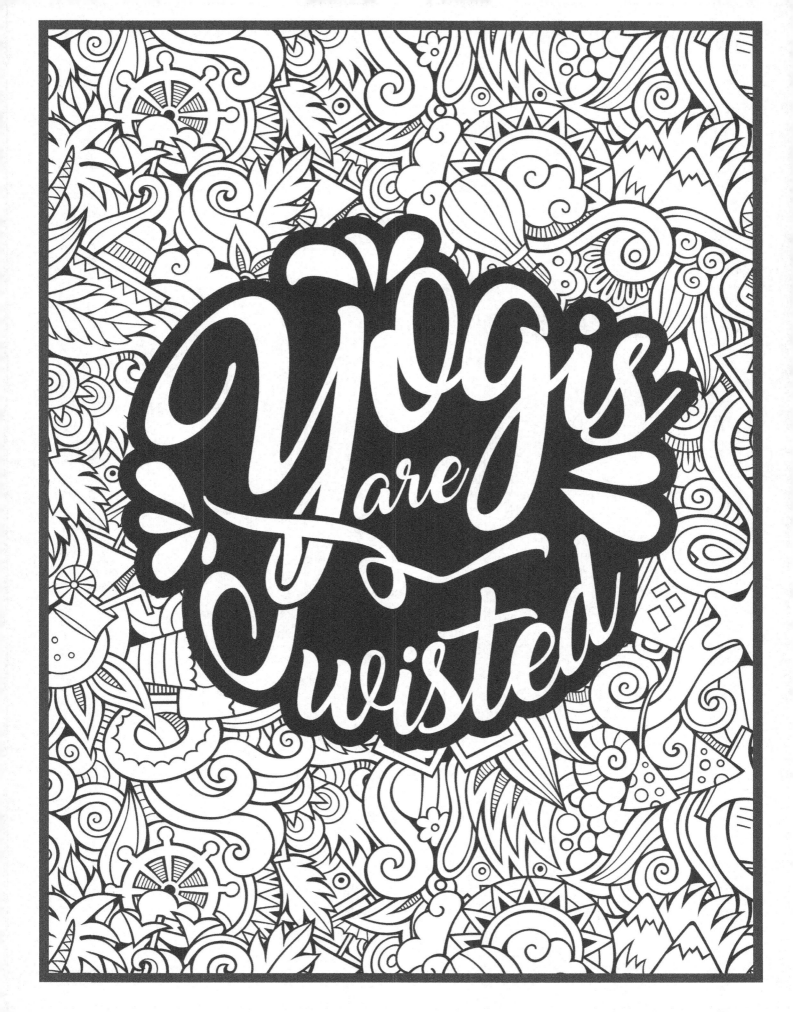

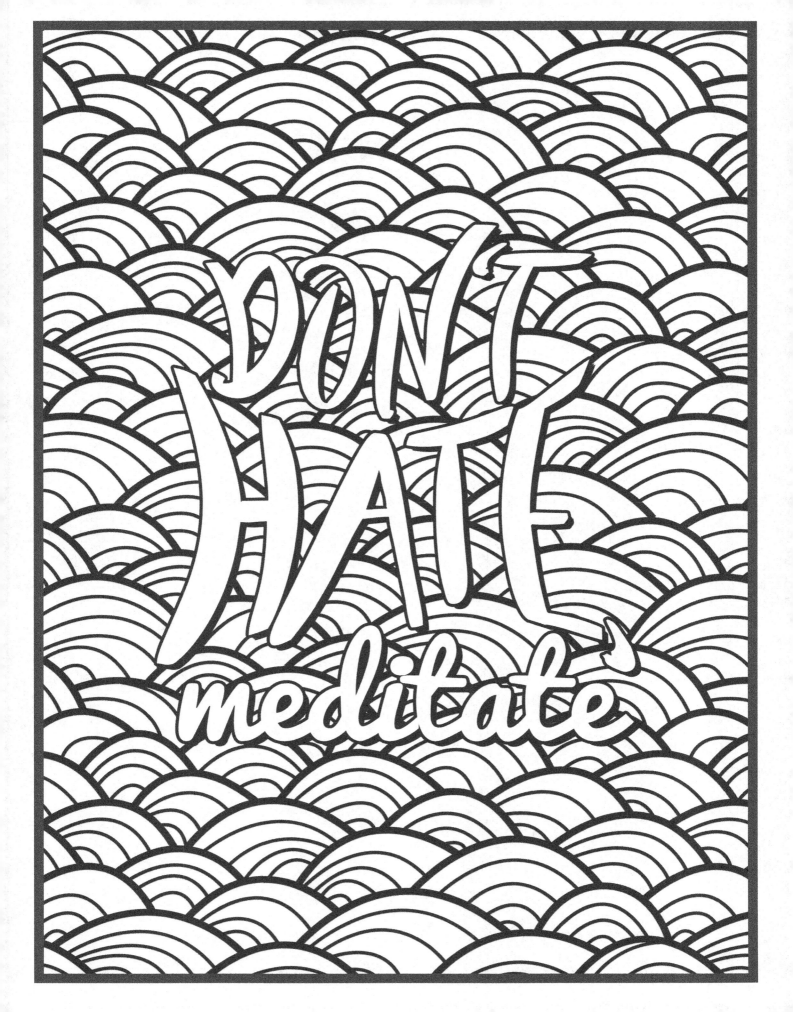

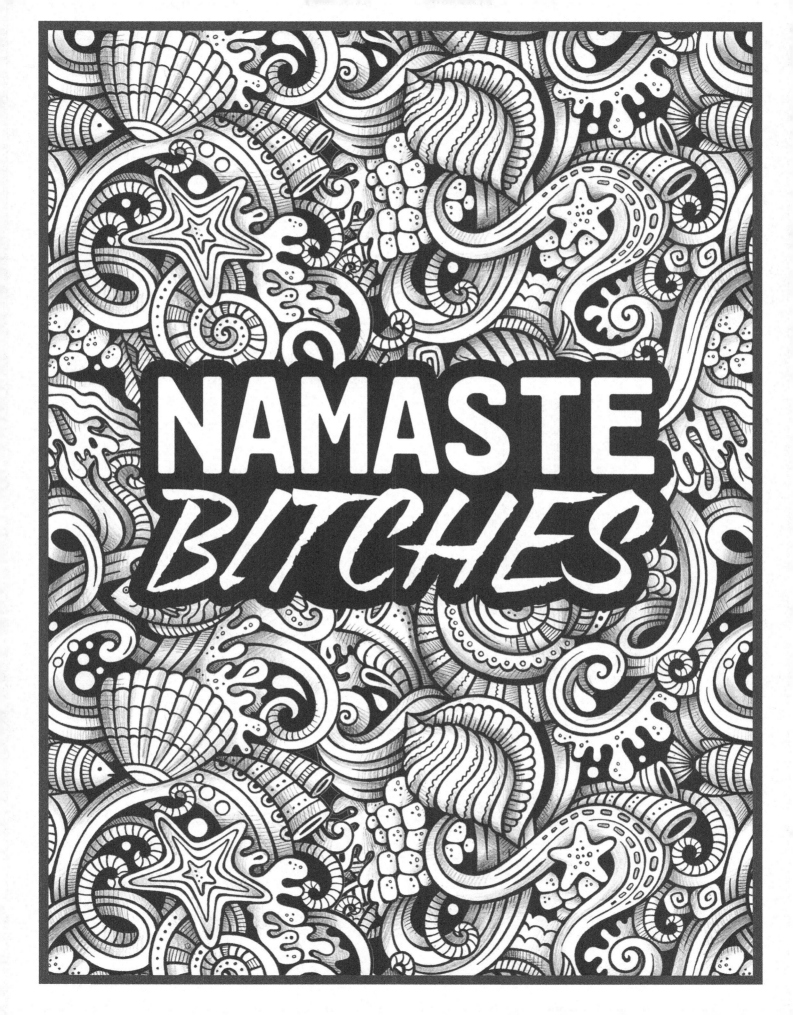

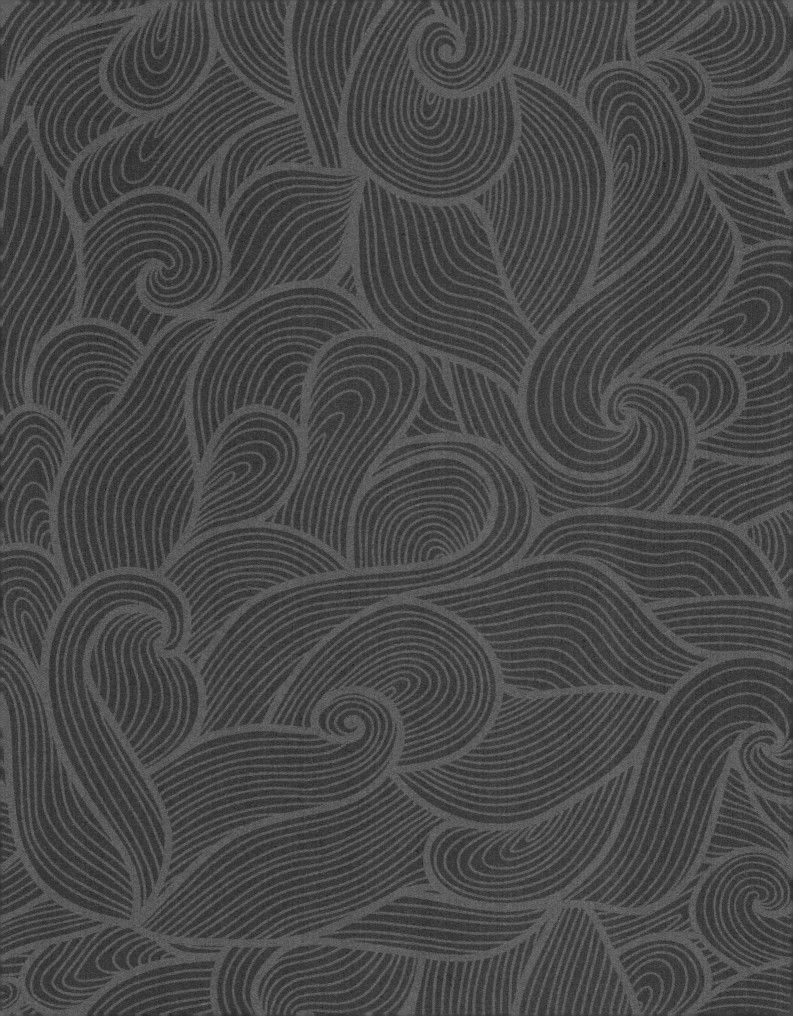

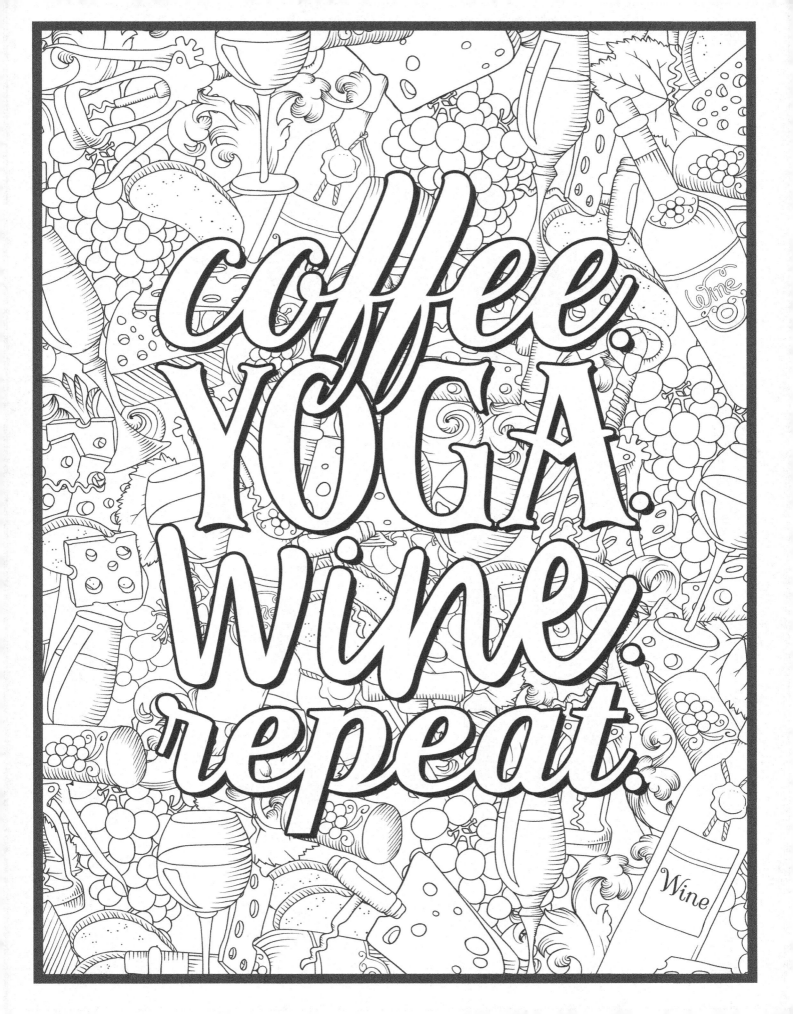

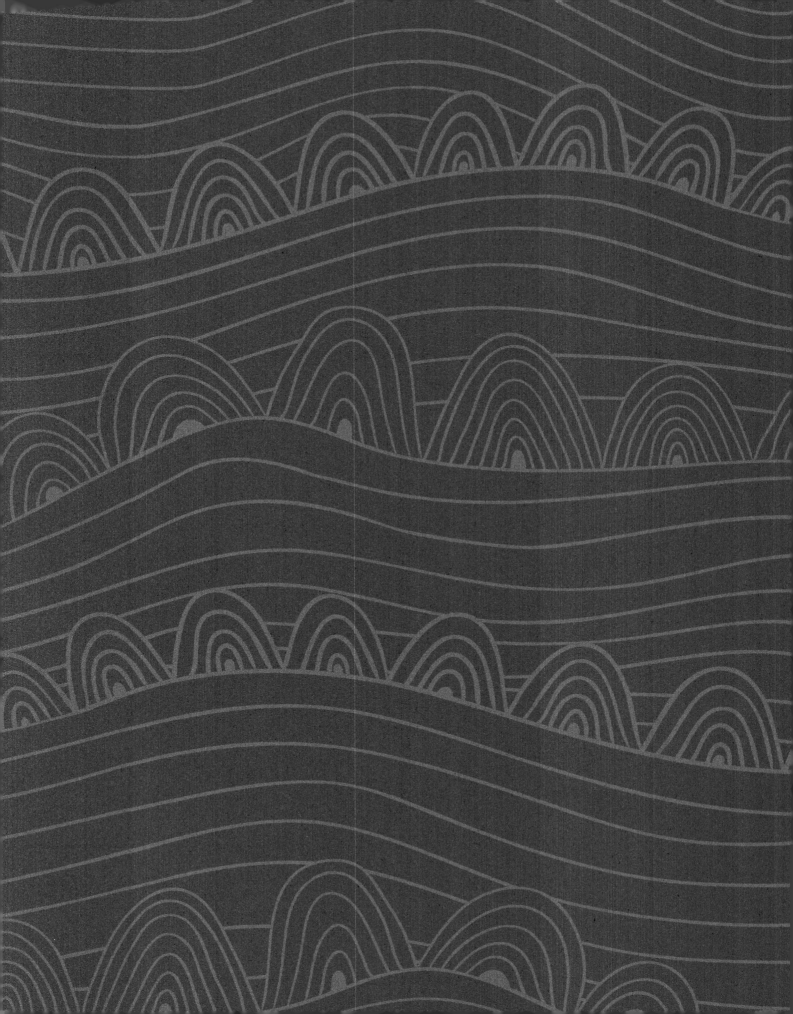

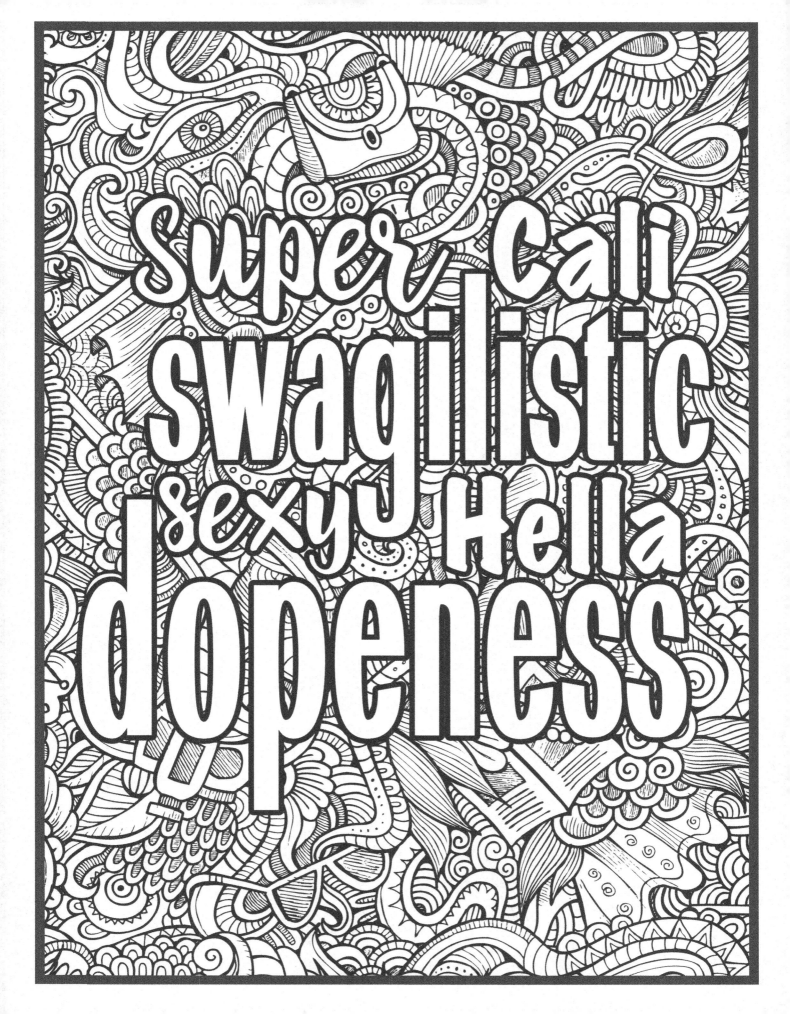

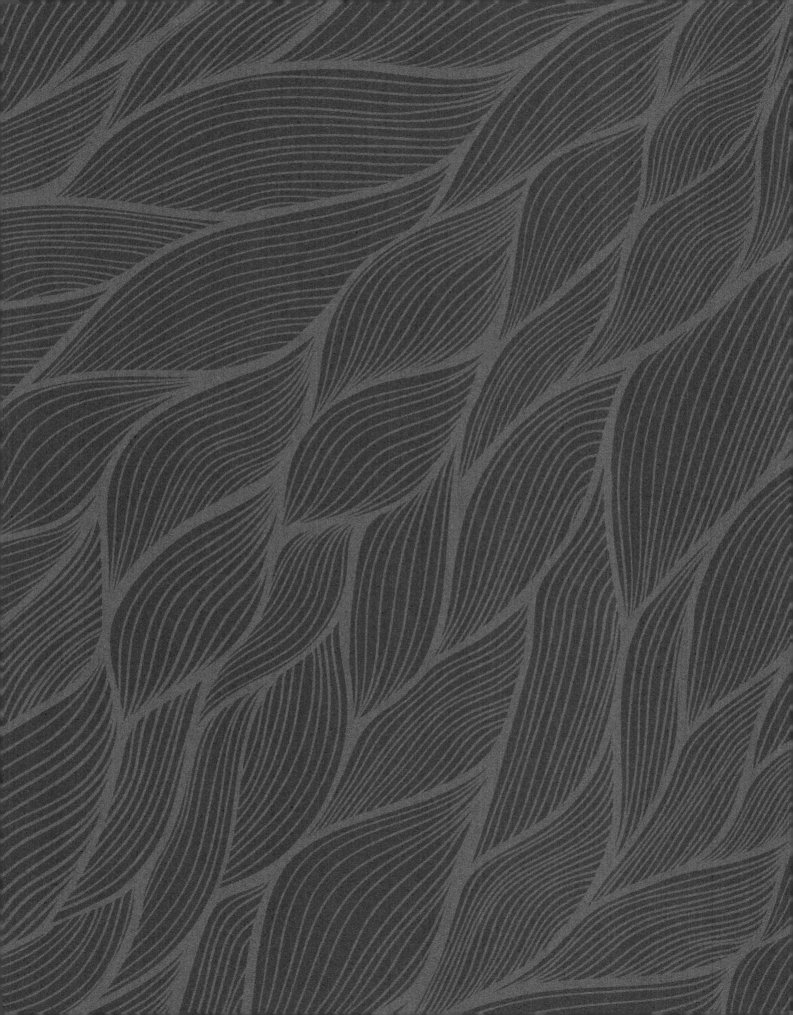

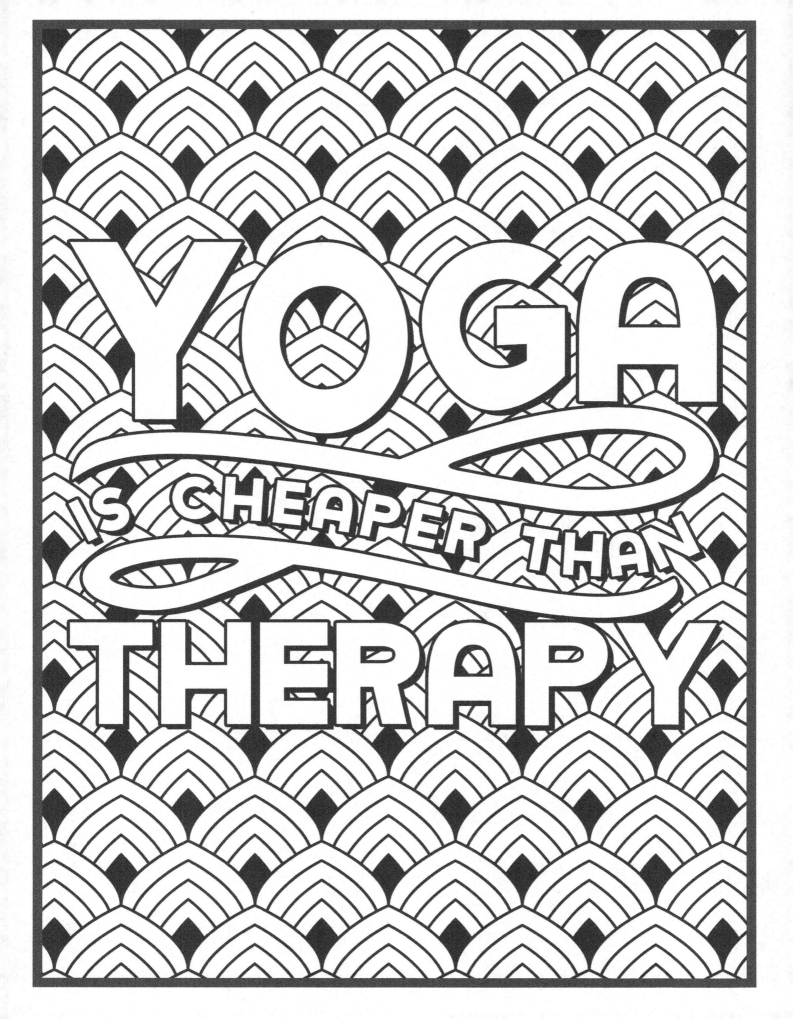

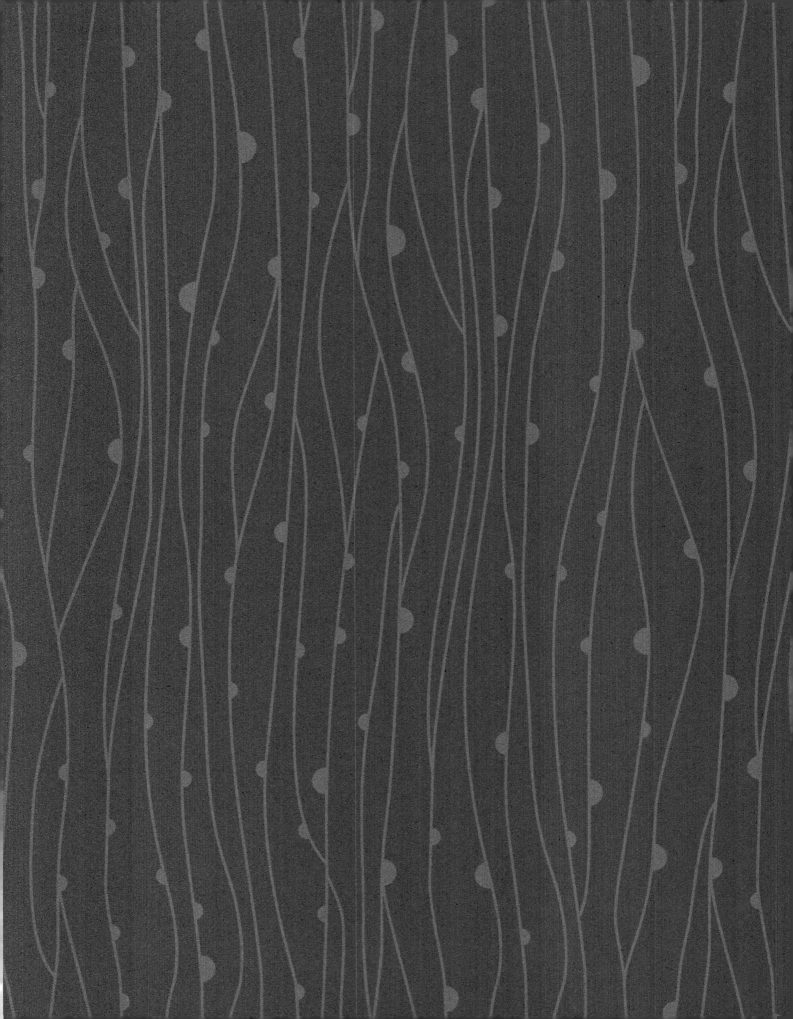

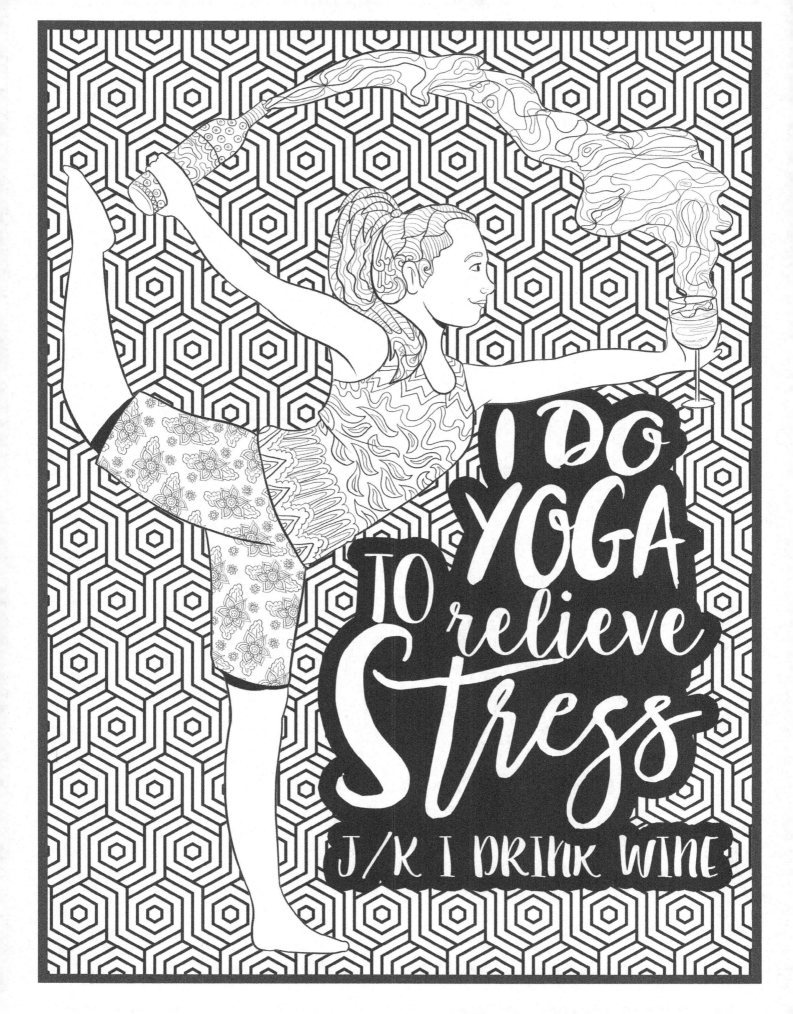

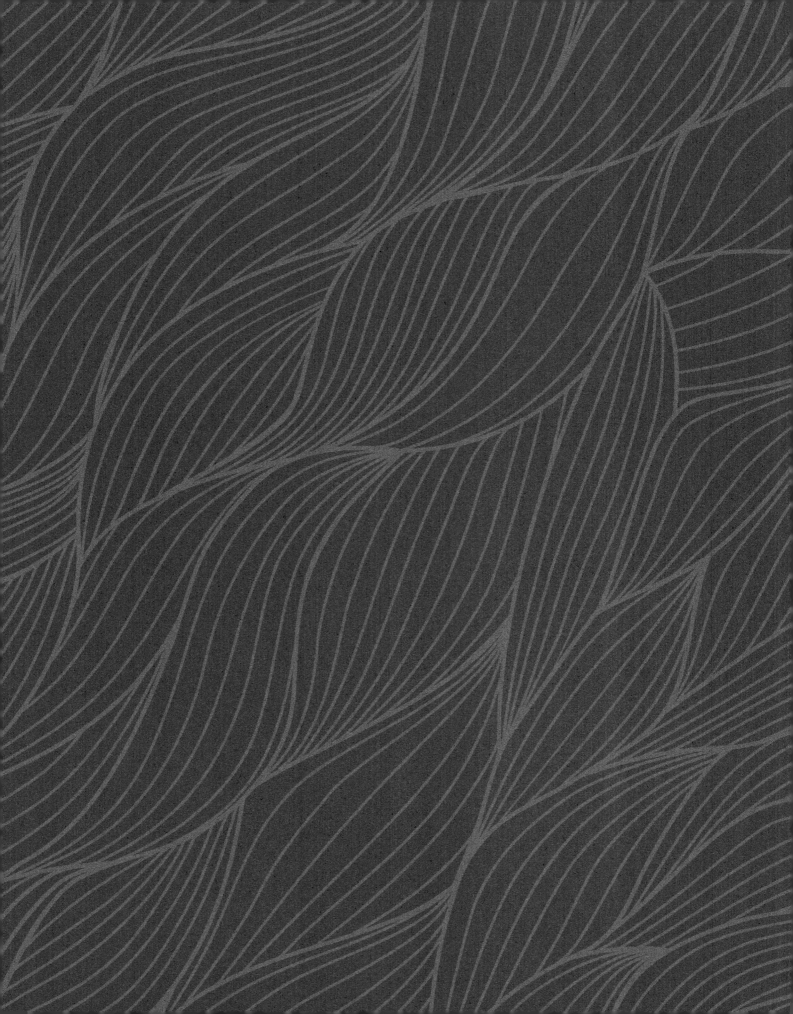

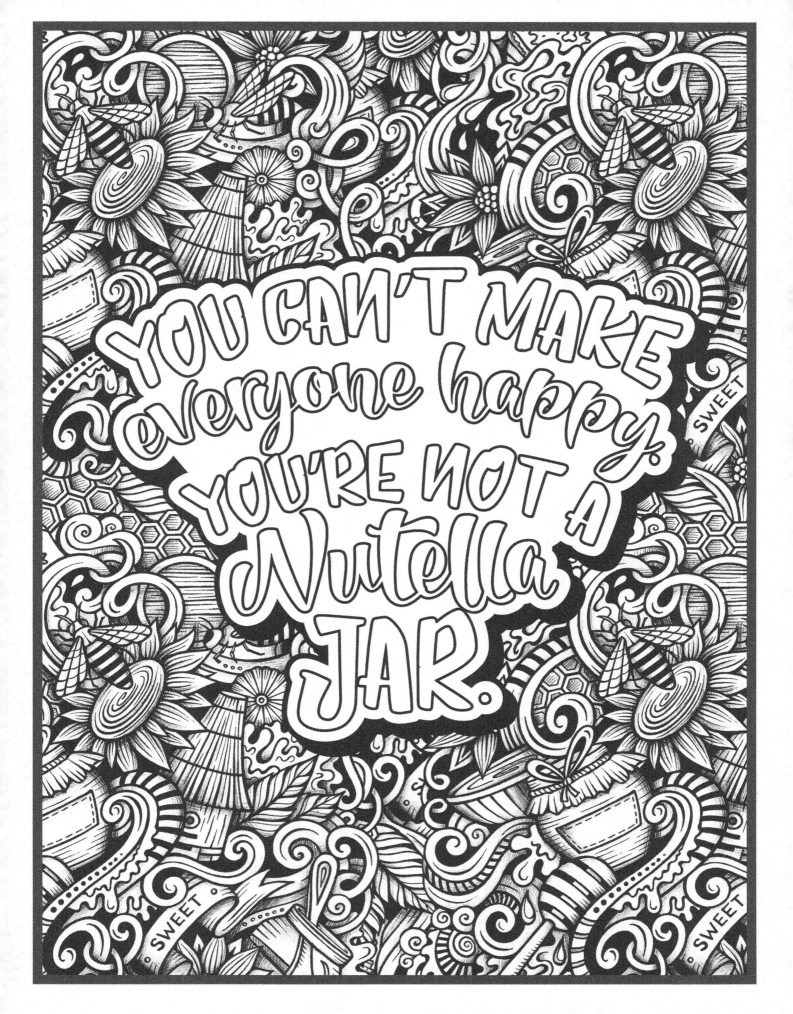

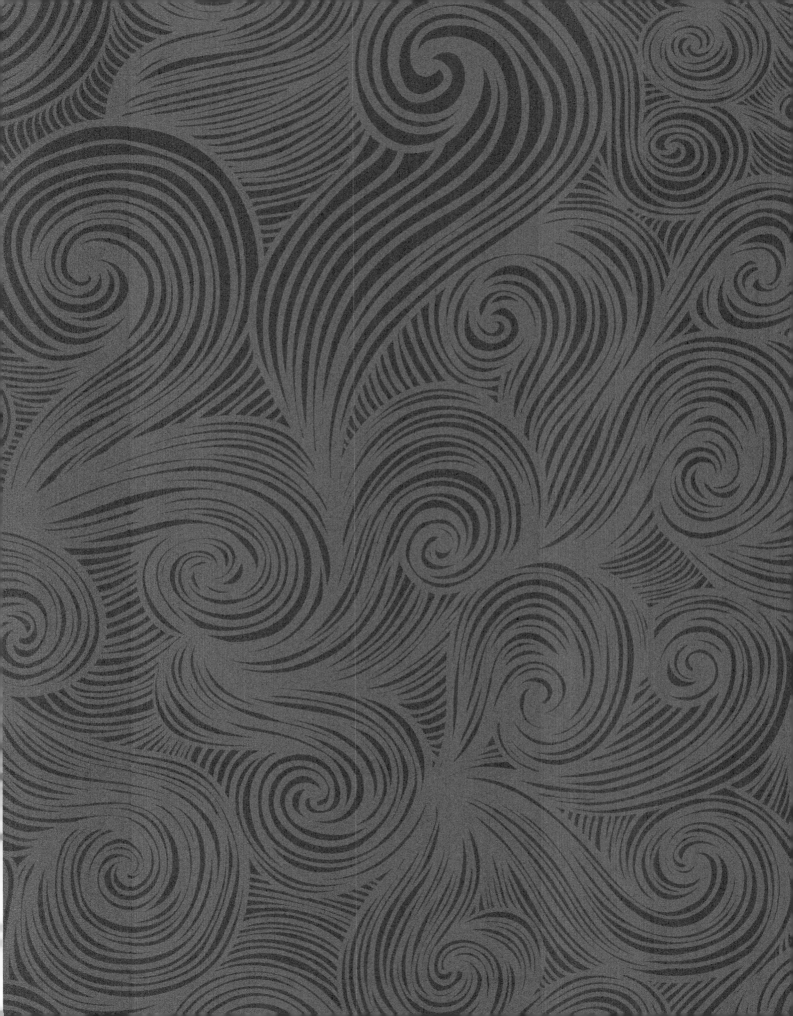

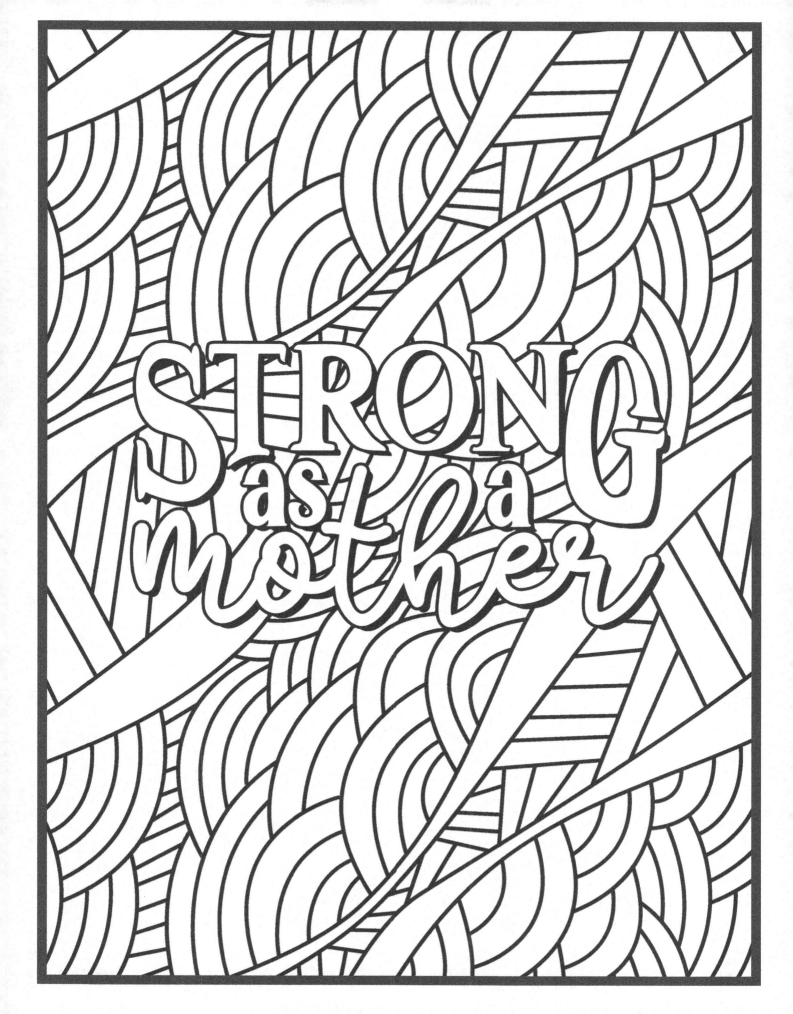

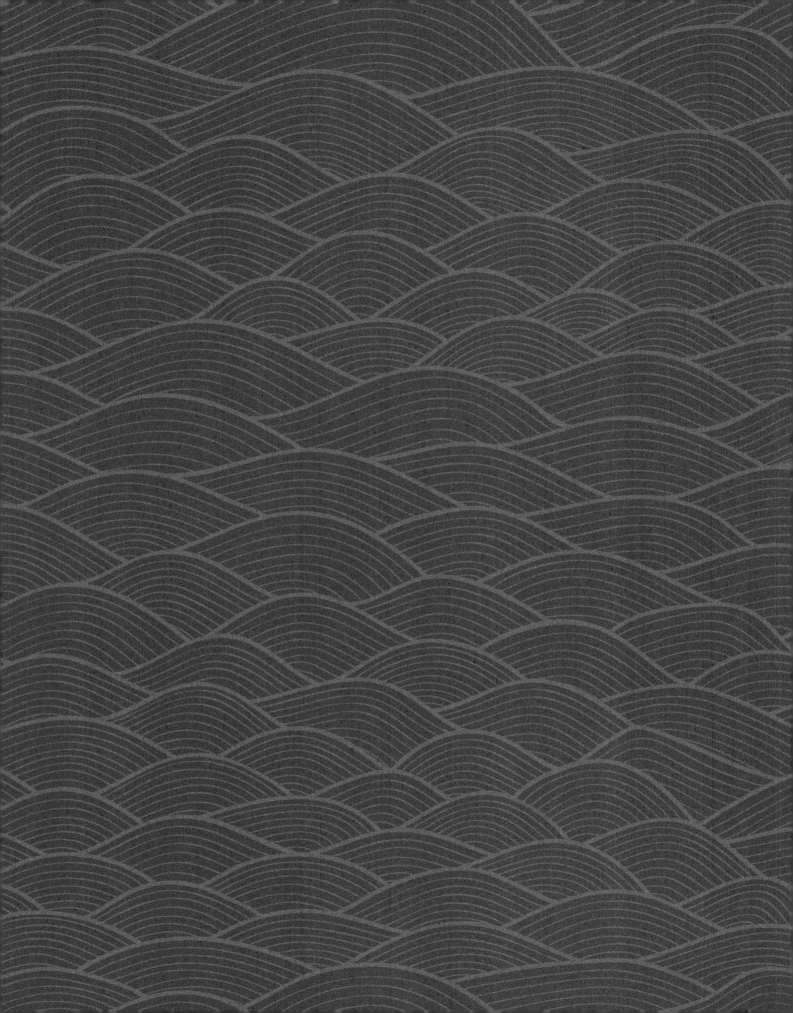

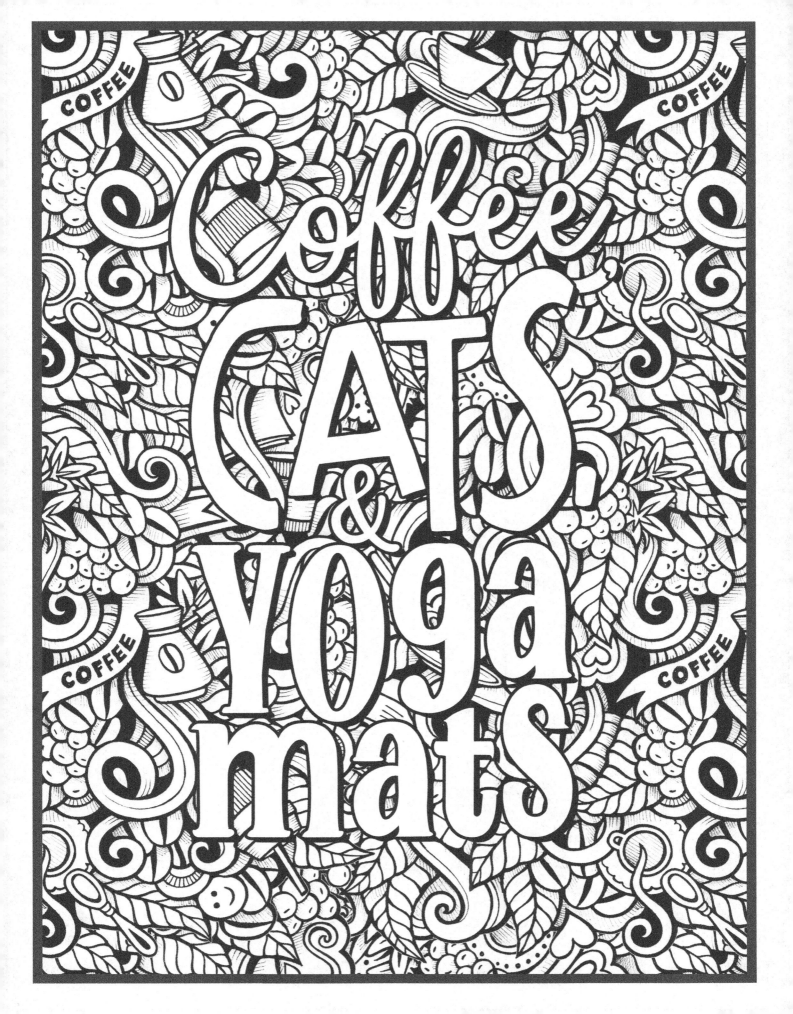

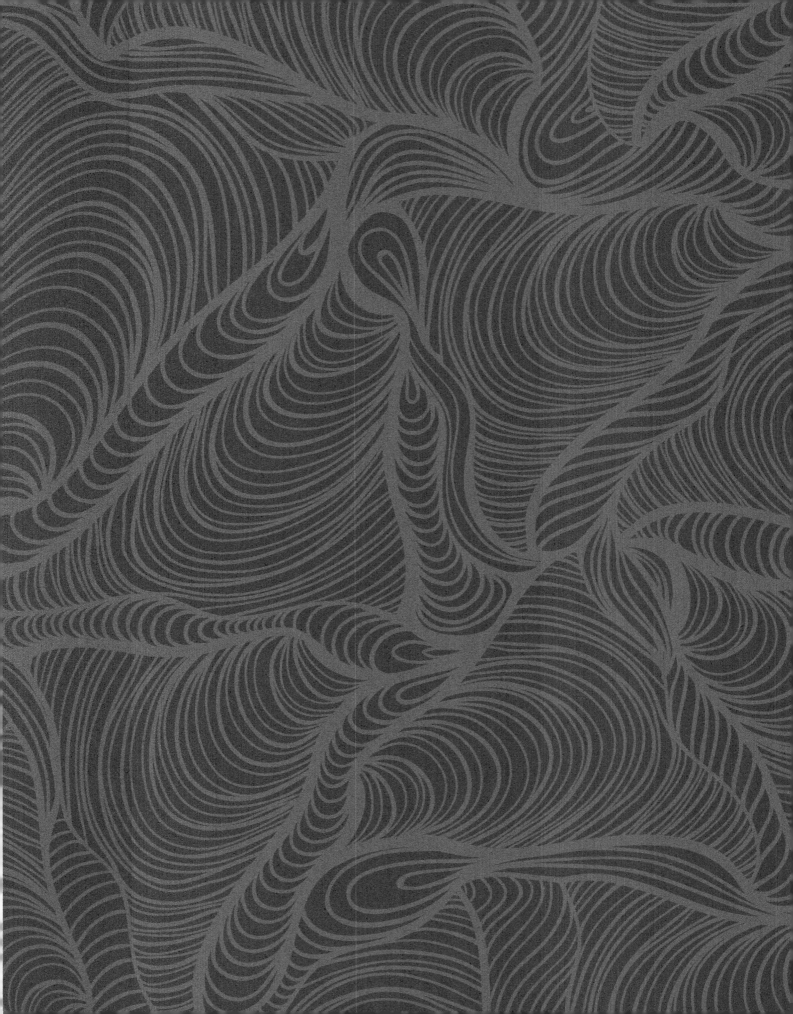

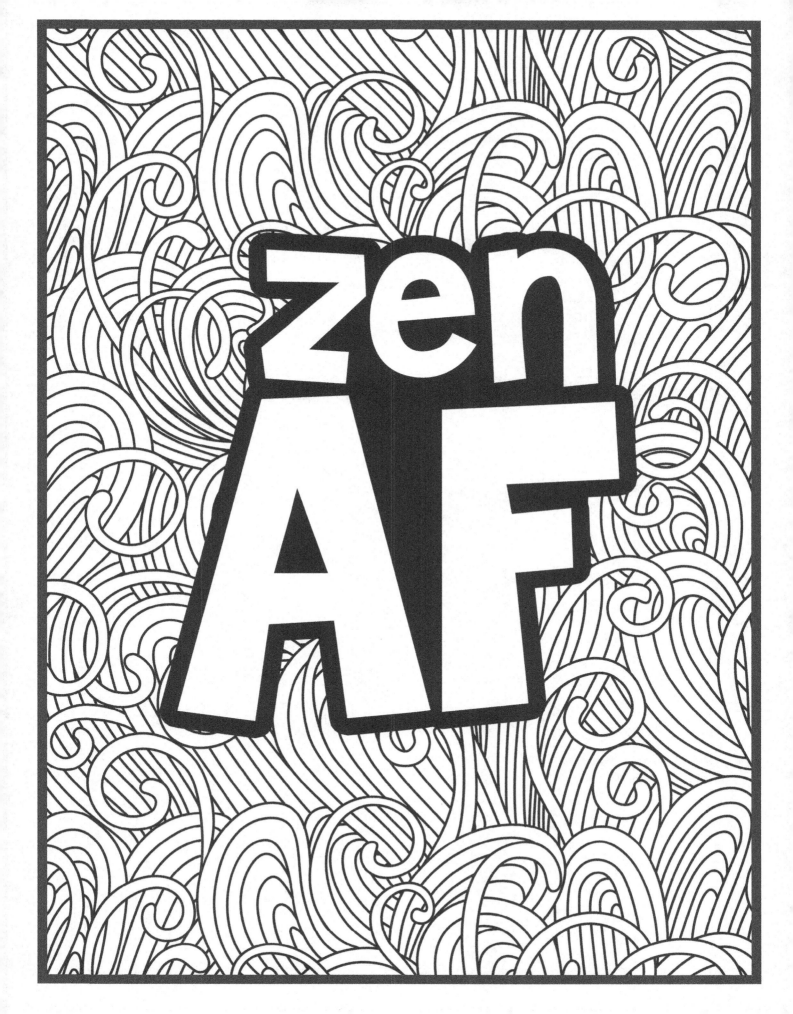

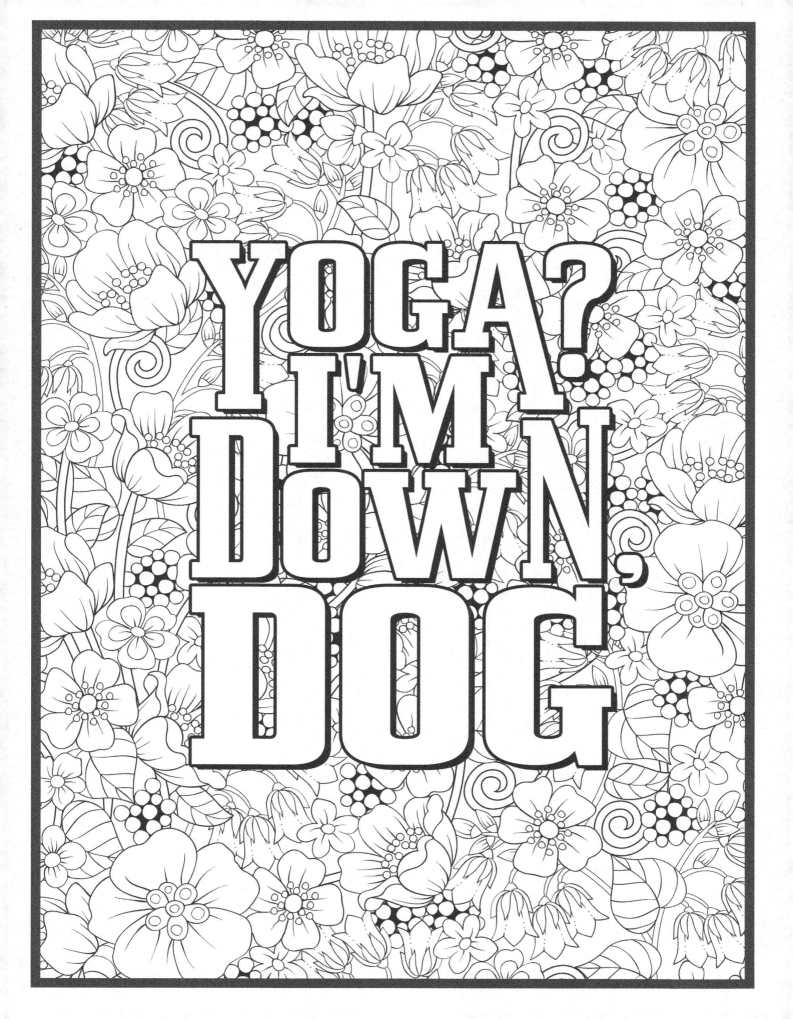

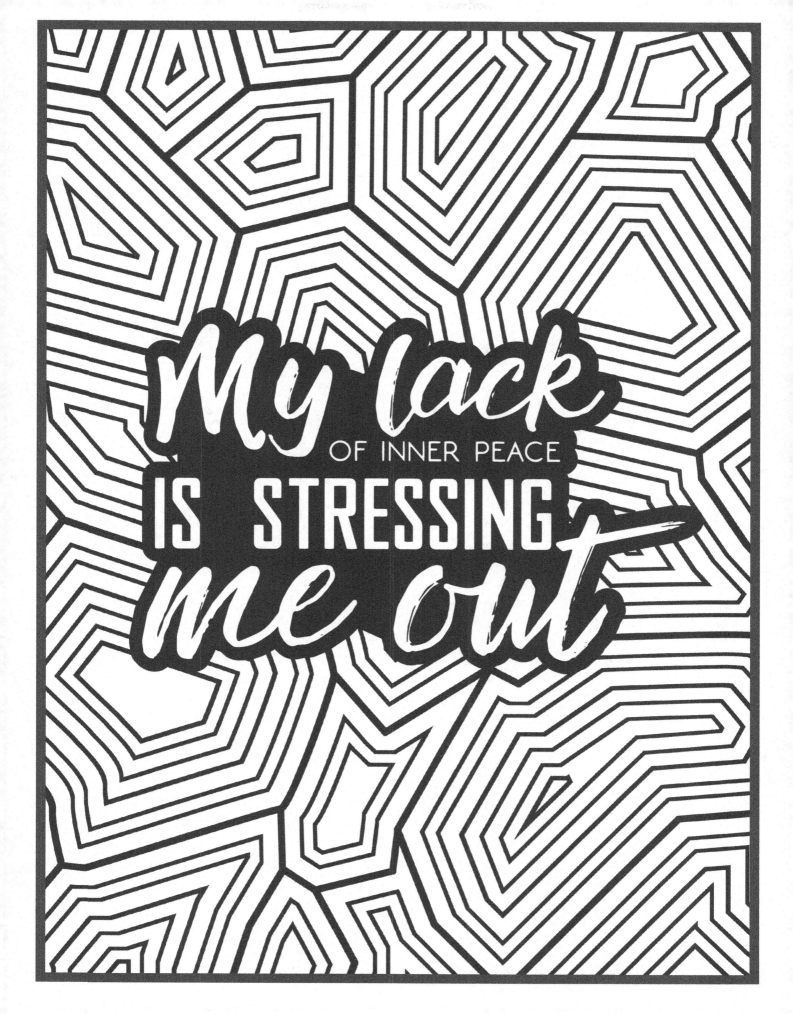

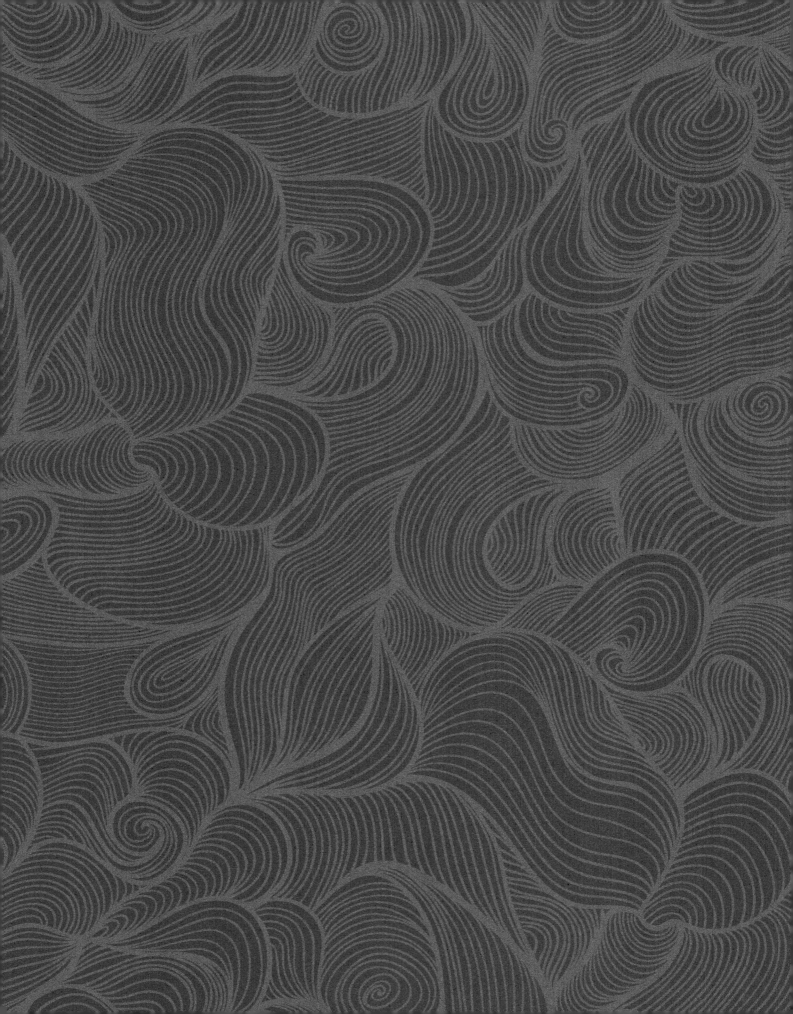

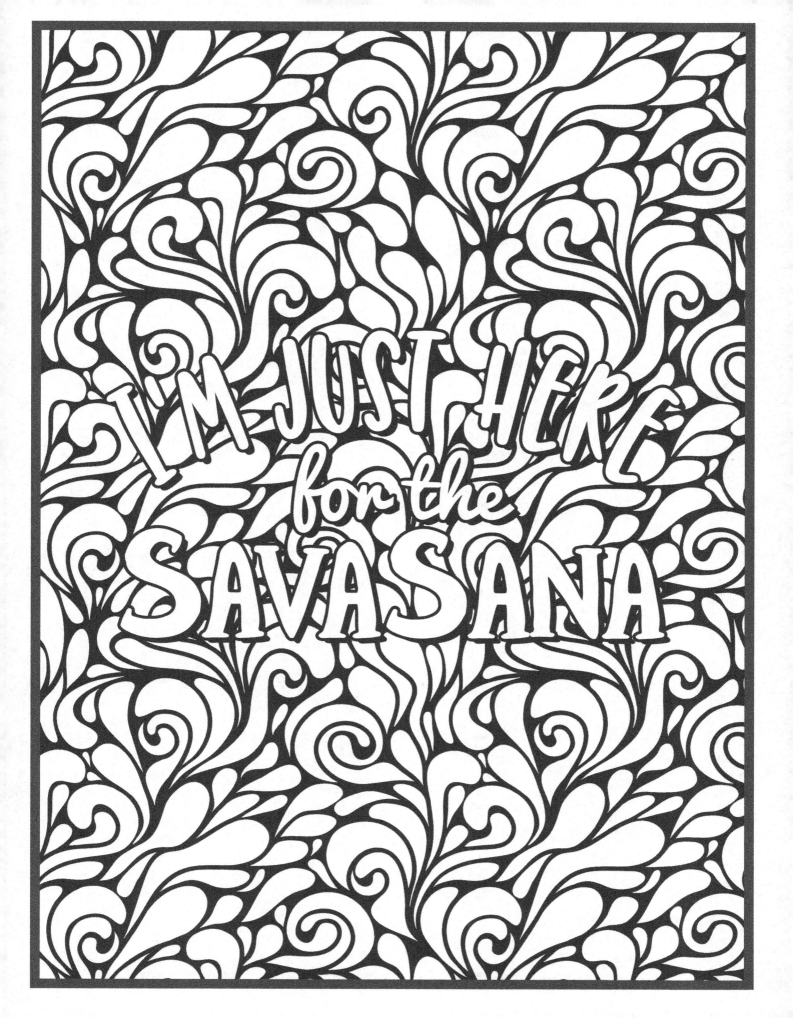

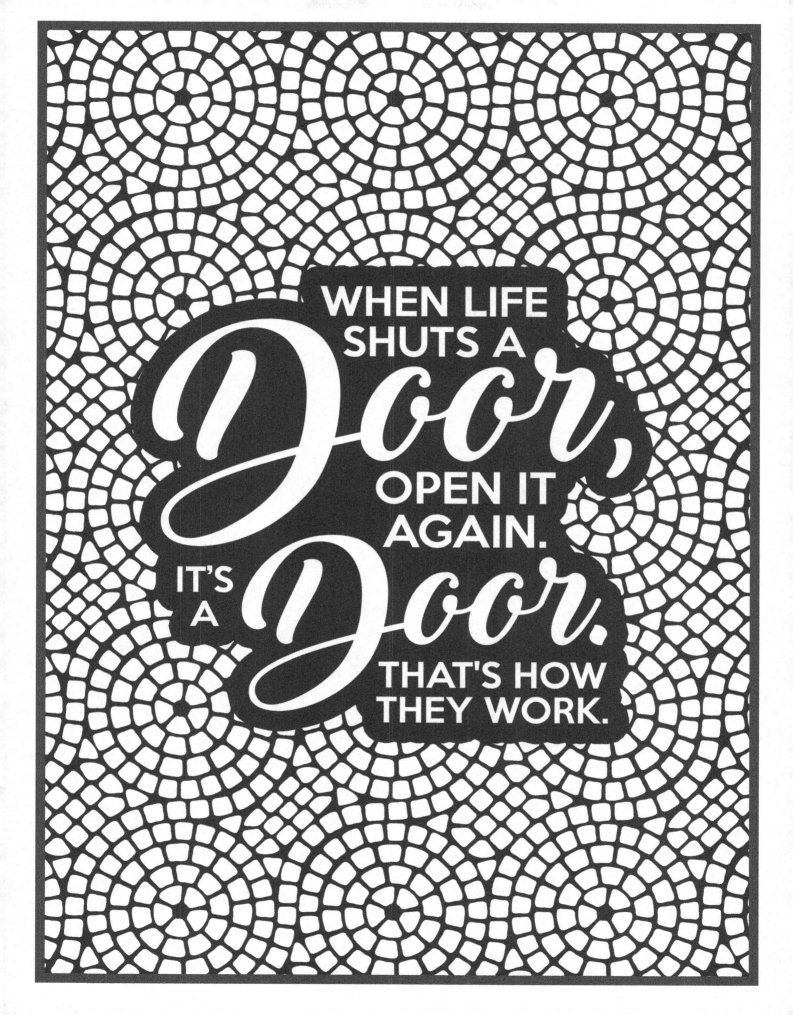

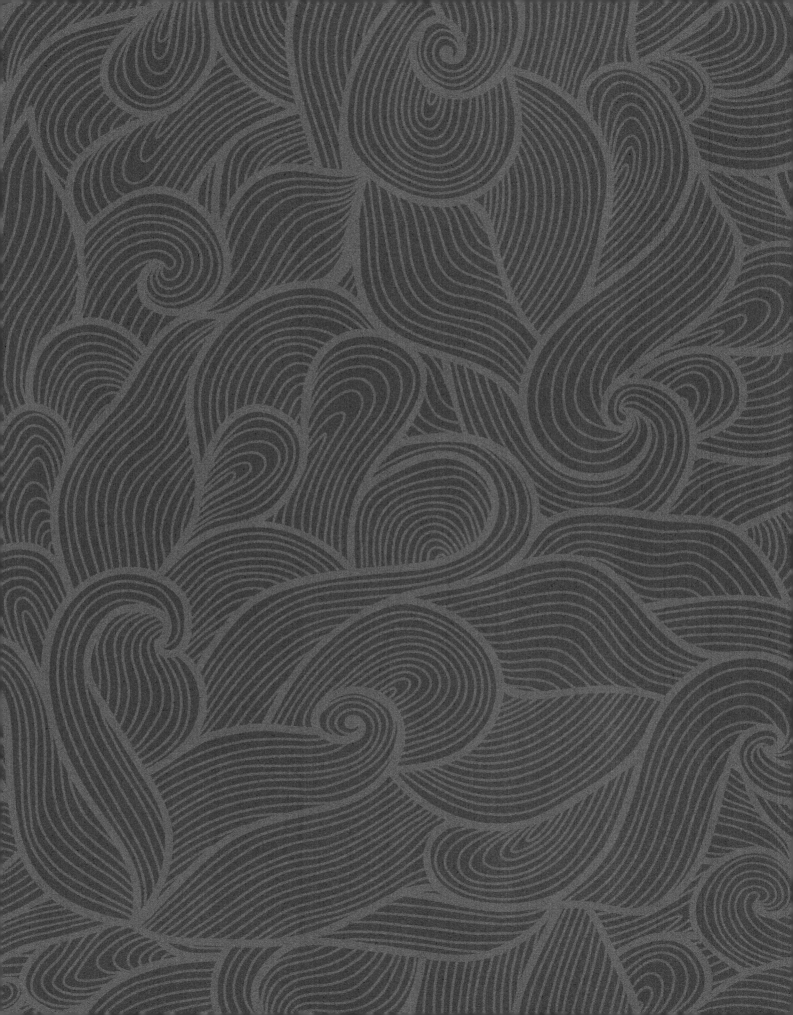